D0907005

THE DESIGN AND MANAGEMENT OF MEDICAL DEVICE CLINICAL TRIALS

THE DESIGN AND MANAGEMENT OF MEDICAL DEVICE CLINICAL TRIALS

STRATEGIES AND CHALLENGES

Salah Abdel-aleem

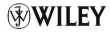

A JOHN WILEY & SONS, INC., PUBLICATION

Published by John Wiley & Sons, Inc., Hoboken, New Jersey.
Published simultaneously in Canada.

For general information on our other products and services or for technical support, please contact our Customer Care Department within the United States at (800) 762-2974, outside the United States at (317) 572-3993 or fax (317) 572-4002.

Wiley also publishes its books in a variety of electronic formats. Some content that appears in print may not be available in electronic formats. For more information about Wiley products, visit our web site at www.wiley.com.

Library of Congress Cataloging-in-Publication Data:

Abdel-aleem, Salah.
   The design and management of medical device clinical trials : strategies and challenges / Salah Abdel-aleem.
      p. ; cm.
   Includes bibliographical references and index.
   ISBN 978-0-470-60225-6 (cloth)
   1. Medical instruments and apparatus–Research.   2. Clinical trials.   I. Title.
   [DNLM: 1. Clinical Trials as Topic–methods.   2. Equipment and Supplies.   3. Device Approval.   W 26 A135d 2010]
   R856.4.A22 2010
   610.28′4072–dc22

                                                                                2009045887

Printed in Singapore

10 9 8 7 6 5 4 3 2 1

For my mother Farha, my loving wife Maro, and my sons Omar, Tarek, and Yussuf. Your support has been truly inspirational.

■■■■■■ CONTENTS

ABR	Angiographic binary restenosis
AE	Adverse event
ARCHeR	ACCULINK for Revascularization of Carotids in High-Risk Patients
BIOMO	Bioresearch monitoring program
BMS	Bare metal stent
BNP	Brain natriuretic peptide
CBER	Center for Biologics Evaluation and Research (FDA)
CDHR	Center for Devices and Radiological Health (FDA)
CDER	Center for Drug Evaluation and Research (FDA)
CEA	Carotid endarterectomy
CE Mark	Mandatory European marking for certain product groups to indicate conformity with the essential health and safety requirements set out in European Directives
CFR	Code of Federal Regulation
CMS	Centers for Medicare and Medicaid Services
COPD	Chronic obstructive pulmonary disease
CRA	Clinical research associate
CRFs	Case report forms
CRO	Clinical research organization
CLI	Critical limb ischemia
DES	Drug-eluting stent
%DS	Percent diameter stenosis
DASI	Duke Activity Status Index Questionnaire
DSMB	Data Safety Monitoring Board
EC	Ethics Committee
ELA	Excimer Laser Atherectomy
EU	European Union
FDA	Food and Drug Administration
LACI	Laser angioplasty for critical limb ischemia
LL	Late loss
GCP	Good clinical practice

HIPAA	Health Insurance Portability Accountability Act
ICD-9	International classification of disease version 9
ICF	Informed consent form
IDE	Investigational device exemption
IND	Investigational new drug
IRB	Institutional review board
ISO	International organization for standardization
ITT	Intent-to-treat analysis
NDA	New drug application
NIH	National Institute of Health
NSR	Nonsignificant risk
MACE	Major adverse cardiac events
MAE	Major adverse event
MEDDEV	Medical device
MedDRA	Medical dictionary for regulatory activities
MLD	Minimum lesion diameter
MI	Myocardial infarction
OHRP	Office of Human Research Protection
OPC	Objective performance criteria
OWR	Over the wire
PAD	Peripheral artery disease
PI	Principal investigator
PMA	Premarket approval
PP	Per-protocol analysis
PSA	Prostate-specific antigen
PTA	Percutaneous transluminal angioplasty
RCT	Randomized controlled trial
RX ACCULINK	Rapid exchange ACCULINK stent
SAP	Statistical analysis plan
SAPPHIRE	Stenting and Angioplasty with Protection in Patients at High Risk for Endarterectomy
SFA	Superficial femoral artery
SES	Sirolimus-eluting stent
SR	Significant risk
RVD	Reference vessel diameter
TAH	Total artificial heart
TASC	Transatlantic Inner Societal Consensus
TLF	Target lesion failure
TLR	Target lesion revascularization
TVR	Target vessel revascularization
UADE	Unanticipated adverse device effect
WHC	Weighted historic control
WHO	World Health Organization

This is the second book in the series Design, Execution, and Management of Medical Device Clinical Trials published in 2009. The first book of this series covered the fundamental basic tasks and activities required for clinical studies, including development of clinical protocol and other clinical materials, selection of investigators and study sites, adverse event definition and reporting, study statistical analysis plan and final clinical protocol, regulations of medical devices, investigator-initiated clinical studies, and basics of the bioethical rules governing clinical trials. The current book is entirely devoted to the challenging issues on the design and management of clinical studies, including the design of the clinical protocol, execution of study, and management of the trial. The design of clinical protocols involves such issues as patient recruitment, investigator and study site selection, and study endpoint determination all of which are addressed in this book. Management of the clinical trial involves resolving compliance issues and missing trial data, for example, and these issues are also addressed. This book provides an in-depth analysis of clinical trials whose primary focus is the medical device, but the design and management applications are also applicable to drug studies. In effect the book should benefit all people who work in clinical research, specifically clinical scientists, clinical managers, biostatisticians, clinical research associates, data management personnel, investigators, and clinical coordinators. The book can also be used as a reference manual for undergraduate and graduate students who are completing their degree in clinical research. The book's in-depth and broad coverage of the challenges facing clinical research makes it particularly useful as a training manuals.

The key lessons of this book can be summarized as follows:

- Coaching on the design of clinical study protocol, including on the selection of sites for complex trials, selection of study endpoints, issues involved in research contract agreements, and the informed consent letter.

- Coaching on managing clinical trials, including slow study enrollment, missing data analysis, protocol deviations, and identification/reporting of adverse events.
- Coaching on the selection of historic controls instead of an active control group in clinical trials.
- Instructions on how to recognize and avoid fraud and misconduct in clinical trials.
- Discussion of the regulations of medical devices, including 510(K) determination, determination of significant and nonsignificant risk devices, and similarities/differences of regulations between drugs and medical devices.
- Review of the CE mark standard of the European Union and other global clinical standards.
- Discussion of high profile FDA PMA cases where unconventional endpoints were used as the primary objectives of the studies.

The reader will learn from this book all the challenges associated with clinical studies and how to deal effectively with clinical research obstacles. Further the reader will learn how to deal effectively with international and global clinical issues. An entire chapter is devoted to understanding CE marking. In this chapter tips are given on how to perform and manage global clinical trials. The discussion of global clinical trials includes FDA criteria for selecting foreign sites.

Further an entire chapter was devoted to high profile FDA PMA cases where unconventional endpoints were used as the primary objectives. For example, the use of subjective endpoint such as improvement of angina class was utilized for the FDA TMR study (transmyocardial laser revascularization). In coronary drug eluting stents, an angiographic late loss, a surrogate endpoint, was used as the primary endpoint. The steps taken by the sponsors of these studies are discussed to show how the endpoints were determined and bias eliminated.

Last the book is intended to provide valuable guidelines on the challenges of clinical studies for clinical scientists (biostatisticians and clinical data analysis experts) who develop and execute scientific clinical tasks, and their research associates. The examples of clinical protocols, statistical analysis plan (SAP), final clinical protocol reports, and the like serve the clinical operational purpose of this book. It is important to recognize that these where these examples employ statistical measures, they are meant to demonstrate the operational purpose of clinical trial data. Taking the operational point of view of clinical challenges can help one better understand the management of trials. With every set of challenges there are presented recommendations on how to deal effectively with those challenges, for example, on the justification of and the parameter settings for the selected historic control.

In summary, this book is intended to be of value to the clinical scientist faced with challenging issues of the design, execution, and management of a trial and looking for practical recommendations on how to deal effectively with these challenges.

SALAH ABDEL-ALEEM, PHD
Senior Clinical Operation Manager
Proteus Biomedical, Inc.

◼️◼️ ACKNOWLEDGMENTS

I would not have been able to write this book without the collaboration of the following wonderful professors and mentors: Professor M. El-Merzabani at the Egyptian National Cancer Institute, who taught me the principles of laboratory research after my graduating from college; Professor Horst Schulz of the City University of New York, my PhD supervisor; Professor James E. Lowe, at Duke University Medical Center, with whom I collaborated for eight years in cardiovascular research; Professor Daniel Burkhoff, at Columbia University, with whom I have collaborated for the past 10 years on clinical research; Professor William Gray, at Columbia University, who provided me with invaluable insight on clinical studies; Professor Ismail Sallam, the former Egyptian Minister of Health, who provided me with insight into international clinical trials; my colleagues at Proteus Biomedical Inc., particularly Dr. Greg Moon, Dr. George Savage, and Dr. Allison Intondi. Also I am appreciative of assistance of my son Omar Abdel-aleem in helping me prepare this book for publication.

Challenges to the Design of Clinical Study

*The Design and Management of Medical Device Clinical Trials: Strategies and
Challenges*, by Salah Abdel-aleem
Copyright © 2010 John Wiley & Sons, Inc.

In today's market the medical device and pharmaceutical industry is facing a number of challenges. The challenges range from the design and management of the study to preparation of clinical trials, and complying with increasingly stringent new regulatory guidelines. As a result these companies must look for efficiencies, faster time to market, and means of reducing costs. In addition, the companies must quickly update their processes and polices to meet the requirements of new standards.

This chapter provides an overview of the preparation and design aspects of clinical trials for medical devices. Upon completion of this chapter, readers will have an understanding of the unique challenges faced in clinical trials for medical devices and will be able to deal effectively with these challenges. This chapter will review challenges, roles, and responsibilities of sponsors and investigators during the clinical development phase.

Challenges to the design of clinical studies are discussed in detail in this chapter. In alliance with the theme of this book, these challenges are discussed from the clinical operational point of view to allow reader to identify and deal with these challenges in an effective and practical manner. Several challenges of the design of clinical trials exist, including the selection of study investigators, study centers, and the appropriate patient population. The selection of investigators, particularly for complex studies or studies where subject enrollment is proceeding at slow rate, is addressed in this chapter.

Challenges of the clinical protocol pertaining to the development of clinical standard operating procedures (SOPs) (to ensure compliance to regulatory guidelines), research contract (particularly subject injury, publication review, and trial timeline), definition of enrolled subject and special problems associated with expected slow enrollment, definition of investigational system and its accessories in the trial, design of the statistical analysis plan (SAP), and selection of study endpoints—primary, secondary, and other endpoints in the study and sample size estimation—are discussed from the operational point view, and recommendations are provided for dealing with these challenges. It should be noted that this book is not meant to be statistical text; an in-depth study of statistical issues is beyond the scope of this book. An SAP should be developed during the early preparation of study, to specify the sample size of the study, study endpoints, and definition of success or failure of the study. The SAP is usually discussed with the FDA during the early phase of the trial. Other important issues in the design of the study such determination of subgroups and subgroup analysis, discussion of superiority versus noninferiority study are also discussed.

Challenges of the development of informed consent form, particularly challenges to the readability, comprehension, and issues regarding the signature of the form are discussed in this chapter. Criteria for review of literature and laying out the background of the study are presented. The elements of the process of risk/benefit analysis of the study are discussed, including risks due to disease, risks due to alternative therapies, risks due to investigational product, mitigation of risks, and the overall risk/benefit assessment.

A set of recommendations were given on how to prepare the review of literature section, selecting the study endpoints, writing the components of an SAP, determining the responsibilities of clinical personnel in completing the study, changing the primary endpoint during the course of the trial, selecting surrogate endpoints, and making the ICF easily readable and more comprehensive.

DEVELOPMENT OF CLINICAL SOPs

One of the important earlier best clinical practices is to develop clinical SOPs (standard operating procedures) to ensure that:

- The sponsor of the studies have consistent processes that meet or even exceed regulatory and good clinical practice (GCP) standards.
- The clinical research staff is familiar with these processes, and the processes are reviewed and updated on a regular basis.
- Audits by the FDA do not result in serious findings.

At a minimum, certain SOPs should be developed prior to the design and execution of clinical studies, such as reporting of adverse events, interim monitoring procedures, development of the ICF template, development of the clinical protocol, and management of clinical file contents.

SELECTION OF STUDY PATIENTS, INVESTIGATORS, AND STUDY SITES

Patient Selection

Patient selection for a clinical study is usually determined by setting up specific inclusion and exclusion criteria for the study. However, patient selection for particular studies sometime becomes a challenge, particularly where enrollment into the trial is extremely slow. Other issues may include a wide or specific selection across a certain disease or disorder. In other words, a balance should be maintained in recruiting patients between being too specific and too diffuse, or the risk of having too narrow inclusion/exclusion criteria versus too wide criteria. An example is presented using the condition of cardiogenic shock. Cardiogenic shock is defined by sustained hypotension with tissue hypoperfusion. Patients presented with this condition based on two different etiologies: ischemic heart disease or mechanical cardiogenic shock (e.g., cardiomyopathies or cardiac valve problems). One advantage of selecting patient with same etiology is the homogeneity of selected patient population and its relation to achieving the study endpoints. A major disadvantage of this selection is the limitation of patient enrollment, and thus limitation of the therapy upon approval to the selected patient population. Part of the response to this challenge is to widely select patients for the feasibility study(s), then tuning up the patient selection to the desired patient population during the pivotal trial. It is always challenging to bring the right balance among selected patients, achievement of the study endpoints, and marketing the product to those selected patients. In general, a tight relationship should be maintained among the selected patient population, study endpoints, and indication for use. Specific inclusion/exclusion criteria of the study are developed to select a particular patient population and ensure protocol selection criteria.

If patients with certain criteria are excluded from the study, then measurements should be provided to ensure the inclusion or exclusion of these patients. For example, if pregnant women are excluded from participating in the study, then negative pregnancy test should be the criterion for all females with child-bearing potential who are enrolled in the study. If patients with renal failure, liver dysfunction, were excluded from participation in the study then tests that evaluate these organ functional statuses and the specific level of parameters that define organ failure should be administered to ensure the exclusion of those patients.

Patient Screening Log

The creation of a patient screening log in a clinical study is important because it defines the criteria for screen failure subjects not being enrolled in the study. This information can be utilized, upon modifying certain criteria, to increase subject enrollment if the enrollment is slow in the trial (see the discussion in Chapter 2 on relaxing study criteria).

The screening log could also be helpful in documenting patient selection criteria for future clinical studies. This log lists all screened subjects, including screen failure subjects, and records why certain subjects were not enrolled in the study. This log serves as proof that an unbiased adequate number of suitable subjects were selected as defined in the protocol. This log contains the following items:

- Site ID number
- Patient ID number
- Did patient meet inclusion/exclusion and baseline assessment criteria? (Yes or No)
- Did patient enroll in the study? (Yes or No)
- Reason why patient is not enrolled in the study
- Date of enrollment if subject is enrolled in the study

Selection of Investigators and Study Sites

The selection of investigators and clinical sites is one of the important steps for preparation of clinical studies. Investigators are usually selected based on their clinical research experience, interest in the proposed study, and the ability to recruit study patients within the proposed duration of the study. The advantages of selecting private hospitals, private practice physicians, or managed care organizations over academic hospital is the reduction of the review time of the application, contract, or IRB approval from approximately 60 to 150 days to 15 to 60 days. Another advantage is the reduction of the overhead cost required by academic institutions. However, a clear advantage of academic institutions is that it has the appropriate facility, experienced investigators, and staff to conduct complex clinical trials that include surgery.

The study sponsor is responsible for selecting the investigators of a clinical study. The qualification and selection of clinical investigators and of study sites are among the early preparatory activities for a study. As mentioned above, the objective is to find investigators who are medically qualified and have previous clinical research experience, strong interest in participating in the study, and the potential to execute the trial as planned. Previous clinical research experience may ascertained by published clinical research or prior participation in clinical studies. The potential investigator should be able to recruit the desired patient population within the projected time duration for subject enrollment, and should have qualified research team and adequate clinical research facility to carry out the research. The research team should consist of co-investigators and clinical research staff that include clinical research coordinator(s). The research facility should have the required diagnostic labs, imaging labs, space for storage of investigational product/study documents, and adequate monitoring space. The principal investigator (PI) must not be blacklisted by the FDA and preferably have experience in dealing with the FDA warning letters. The PI should also be conversant with IRB regulations. The PI must provide financial disclosure to the sponsor in accordance with the FDA regulations. A list of potential investigators could be obtained from the sales and marketing departments of the sponsor, other investigators, the scientific advisory committee, CRO, and previous publications. The investigators of the study are usually recommended by the sales and marketing group of the sponsor, by other investigators, or through recognition of their published research.

A potential complication in the selection of investigators is that the candidate researcher may be involved in too many studies and not have the time to supervise another study. This issue could be circumvented by finding out during the investigator qualification visit whether the investigator could complete the study within the proposed time? and whether the investigator is engaged in any other competitive studies?

Certain studies necessitate extra requirements in addition to all of the basic points listed above. For example, a clinical trial may require the selection of physicians from several departments to serve the role of principal investigator and provide optimal management of study subjects at the selected site. This set up was proved to be efficient in complex surgical trials, such that call for the use of left ventricular assist devices or percutaneous replacement of heart valves where a team of physicians (e.g., cardiac surgeon, interventional cardiologist, heart failure cardiologist) is selected as the investigative team to implant device and provide optimal management for the patients.

Usually a principal investigator (PI) is selected by the sponsor to serve as the PI of the entire study. This selection is based on the experience, integrity, interest, and leadership of the PI. However, certain complex studies may require the selection of a team of PI investigators. This team should include physicians from different disciplines in accordance with the proposed issues of the study or the subject enrollment in the trial.

Nonmedical Person as the Principal Investigator

Usually a licensed physician or a dentist is selected as the principal investigator at the study site. However, a qualified nonphysician could conduct or supervise the study provided that this accords with the protocol of the study and/or national and local laws. Nevertheless, a physician should serve as subinvestigator or consultant for the study.

DEFINITION OF ENROLLED SUBJECTS IN A CLINICAL STUDY

The definition of "enrolled subjects" depends on the type of clinical trial. In some clinical trials subjects who meet all inclusion/exclusion criteria and have signed the informed consent are considered enrolled. Other trials additionally randomize subjects who meet all the criteria. In certain clinical trials the subject is considered enrolled after the placement of the investigational product, such as in stent clinical studies. It is clear that the definition of enrolled subject can differ from trial to trial, so the exact meaning of this term should be defined in the clinical protocol.

DEFINITION OF THE INVESTIGATIONAL DEVICE SYSTEM

The investigational device should be clearly defined in the protocol. In some studies the investigational device consists of a system made up of the investigational device plus other accessories, which are considered part of the functioning system. In this case the investigational device is the entire system of the device and accessories, even though some of the accessories may be approved devices by the FDA, but how these accessories function within the new system is to be proved.

RESEARCH CONTRACT CHALLENGES

The research contract is a legally binding agreement involving an offer from pharmaceutical/medical device company-sponsor and acceptance by institution and investigator for services and results, or by institution and investigator in exchange for money from sponsor to conduct the research/trial.

The research contract includes the following points:

- Names, titles, and addresses of the parties involved
- Responsibilities of the principal investigator (PI)
- Subject Injury reimbursement plan

- Payments to the clinical sites and the terms of payment
- Schedule of payments
- Deliverables required for payments
- Indemnification
- Publication policy

Contract signing is one of the latest steps in approving clinical studies by clinical sites, and this document is usually executed just prior to initiating the study. Sufficient time should be planned to complete this activity, especially if the selected site is an academic institution because of the time period required to review and sign the contract.

The budget for the research should be appropriately set up to cover the expenses of the research, institution overhead cost, subject reimbursement, administrative cost, and research staff cost. The research expenses should be limited to research procedures that are not covered by the standard of care. For multicenter trials, negotiation with the cost of research procedures starts with the Medicare prices for these procedures. Subject reimbursement includes the cost of travel of the subject and any reimbursement associated with time spent on research activities to provide responses to specific study questionnaires. Institution overhead cost is usually constant and institution dependent. Administrative costs include expenses for advertisement for the study, mail, coping, and other appropriate costs. The IRB cost for the study is usually set up as direct billing from the IRB to the sponsor.

Challenges to the research contract of a clinical study could exist in five categories of the contract:

- Terms and condition of patient enrollment and completion of the study
- Indemnification
- Publication policy
- Insurance
- Subject's injury

Terms and Condition of Patient Enrollment and Completion of the Study

It is recommended that the terms and condition of patient enrollment and study completion be provided in the contract and connected to payment to the site. In addition terms of subject replacement of withdrawn subjects and completion of case report forms should be stated in the contract. Terms of payment to the site by the sponsor should be mentioned in the contract. Payment throughout the study should be discussed in the contract, such as whether 30% or 50% will be paid to the site upon the completion of 50% enrollment.

Indemnification

The contract should specify whether the sponsor will or will not indemnify, or whether the sponsor is requesting mutual indemnification. It is usually stated in the contract that the site will not incur liability by the normal course of business, any provision of service in connection with study, and sponsor's indemnification in case of manufacturing defect of the study product.

Insurance

The sponsor should carry minimum levels of insurance and prove liquid assets to cover liabilities as are mainly determined by the risk of the study.

Publication

The research contract usually allows for 30 to 60 day publication review and may include other terms for publication restriction, or approval.

Subject's Injury

The contract includes a paragraph about subject injury reimbursement that is not related to physician negligence.

REVIEW OF LITERATURE

A critical review of literature should be conducted by the sponsor of the study during the early phases of the preparation of the clinical investigation. This section will serve as the scientific background and rational for the proposed study. The following procedure is recommended for writing this section:

1. The study sponsor should specify the selection criteria for selected publications such as key words used to specify research, articles only written in English, criteria for selecting papers for meta-

analysis studies, source of published or unpublished research including the exact citation and date of publication, and data cited in peer-reviewed journals.

2. The study sponsor should specify the statistical methods of analysis employed and/or methods used to weight the different papers.
3. The review of literature or the background section should include the following subsections:
    a. Background on the disease or condition to be treated, the patient population, the indication of use, and the economic impact of the condition. A discussion of the effect of disease on economy may include the percentage of incidence, severity of disease, and effect of disease on society.
    b. Description of use of the investigational product, similar products, or alternative therapies. The discussion may include a detailed description of investigative product, its intended functions, and its technological features, as well as similar technologies and their intended use. A comparison may be made of the investigative product to an already existing alternative system, including a list of the advantages and disadvantages of the investigational product when compared to the alternative therapies.
    c. A critical review of the risks associated with use of the investigational product and safety measures to mitigate or minimize these risks.
    d. A conclusion with clear justification of the conduct of the proposed research. Ideally evidence should be generated from controlled clinical studies that are cited in peer reviewed journals.

The review of literature is a scientific process, and the sponsor should observe the following:

1. Present the supporting evidence as well as the counteropinions of researchers.
2. When presenting evidence from meta-analysis studies the sponsor should follow a scientific methodology utilized in generating data from these studies such as indication of use, similarity and differences between studies, whether or not these studies were controlled, and whether single or multicenter studies were involved.
3. The weighted evidence derived from the cited literature should support the rational for the proposed studies.

CHALLENGES TO THE DESIGN OF THE STUDY PROTOCOL, STATISTICAL ANALYSIS PLAN (SAP), AND SELECTION OF STUDY ENDPOINTS

Confirmatory trials must have their analyses prespecified in a statistical analysis plan (SAP) and data quality must be assured by well-documented analysis datasets submitted for review to the regulatory body. The protocol of the study must contain sufficient details, clear specifications, and appropriate methodologies for the study endpoints and their determination.

Developing a Statistical Analysis Plan Guidance

Structured Document Template The following is a high-level outline of the SAP:

1 Introduction
2 Study design and objectives
3 General analysis definitions
4 Demographics and baseline characteristics
5 Patient disposition
6 Study medication and concomitant therapy
7 Efficacy analyses
8 Safety analyses
9 Quality of life
10 Pharmacoeconomics
11 Pharmacokinetics and pharmacodynamics
12 Interim analyses and safety monitoring analyses
13 Reference
14 Protocol violations

Sample: Structured Document Template The following is more structured outline of the SAP:

1 Introduction
2 Study design and objectives
   2.1 Study objectives
      2.1.1 Primary objectives
      2.1.2 Secondary objectives

Guidance to Data Listings   Data listings are important items in the SAP and it represent how data listings are organized in various tables, figures, and charts. Individual subject data listings may include:

- Data tabulations
  Data tabulations data sets
  Data definitions
- Data listing
  Data listing data sets
  Data definitions
- Analysis datasets
  Analysis data sets
  Analysis programs
  Data definitions

MASKING OR BLINDING

The following masking or blinding procedures should be specified in the clinical protocol:

- Keep the identity of treatment assignments masked for:
  Subject
  Investigator, treatment team, or evaluator
  Evaluation teams

- Bias reduction is the purpose of masking
    Each group masked eliminates a different source of bias
- Masking is most useful when there is a *subjective* component to treatment or evaluation:
    No blind—all patients know treatment
    Single blind—patient does not know treatment
    Double blind—neither patient nor health care provider know treatment
    Triple blind—patient, physician, and data analysis personnel do not know treatment
- Double blind is recommended when possible:
    Ensures that subjects are similar with regard to post-treatment variables that could affect outcomes
    Minimizes the potential biases resulting from differences in management, treatment, or assessment of patients, or interpretation of results
    Avoids subjective assessment and decisions by knowing treatment assignment
    Ethics: double-masking should not result in any harm or undue risk to a patient
    Practicality: some treatments may be impossible to mask
    Avoidance of bias: masked studies require extra effort (manufacturing look-alike pills, setting up coding systems, etc.)
    Compromise: sometimes partial masking, such as independent masked evaluators, are sufficient to reduce bias in treatment comparison
- Although masked trials require extra effort, sometimes they are the only way to obtain an objective answer to a clinical question.
- Patients on "notreatment" or standard treatment may be discouraged or drop out of the study.
- Patients on the new drug may exhibit a "placebo" effect, meaning the new drug may appear better when it is actually not.
- Subject reporting and cooperation may be biased depending on how the subject feels about the treatment.
- Treatment decisions can be biased by knowledge of the treatment, especially if the treatment team has preconceived ideas about either treatment:
    Dose modifications
    Intensity of patient examination
    Need for additional treatment.

> Influence on patient attitude by enthusiasm shown (or not) regarding the treatment.

- If endpoint is subjective, evaluator bias will lead to recording more favorable responses on the preferred treatment.
- Even supposedly "hard" endpoints often require clinical judgment, such as blood pressure, MI.
- Treatments can be objectively evaluated.
- Recommendations to stop the trial for "ethical" reasons will not be based on personal biases.
- Sometimes triple-mask studies are hard to justify for reasons of safety and ethics.
- A policy not recommended, not required by FDA.

PRIMARY AND SECONDARY OUTCOMES

Both primary and secondary endpoints should be clearly described in the objective section of the trial protocol.[1] Statistical considerations appropriate to the design of the study, including sample-size calculations, timeline for any interim analysis, and a sketch of a proposed statistical plan for analyzing these endpoints, should be described in detail in the statistical section of the protocol.[2] The analysis principle for the primary outcome must be that of intention-to-treat, where the data are analyzed according to the treatment group to which they were randomized.[3]

SELECTION OF STUDY ENDPOINTS

Features and Characteristics of Endpoints

- List endpoints relevant to disease process that are easy to interpret.
- Focus on a single or a limited number of endpoints.
- Base primary endpoint on clinical outcomes of the study or a surrogate endpoint.
- Ensure that endpoint is free from measurement or assessment error.
- Ensure that endpoint is sensitive to treatment differences.
- Keep endpoints measurable within a reasonable period of time.
- Distinguish between primary and secondary endpoints.

What Makes a Good Primary Endpoint?

The following points contribute to the selection of good primary endpoint:

- Endpoint must answer the primary question.
- Frequency of occurrence of treatment must be known in control.
- Treatment effect must have estimable clinical relevance.
- Treatment must be assessed/evaluable in all participants.
- Treatment must be measured accurately/reliably/objectively.

DIFFERENCES BETWEEN THE PRIMARY ENDPOINT IN FDA AND CE MARK STUDIES

The difference in the primary endpoint selection in the FDA pivotal and the CE Mark studies is discussed in Chapter 6, section under "Differences between the Primary Endpoint in the FDA and the CE Mark Studies." In general, to satisfy the European CE marking requirement, the device must be demonstrated to be safe and perform as intended. To market a class III high-risk (and some class II) device in the United States, the device must be demonstated to be reasonably safe and effective. Effectiveness is usually based on proving clinical outcome in a study.

SAP AND STUDY ENDPOINTS

Key components of the statistical analysis plan for the primary endpoint or endpoints include the specification of how the outcome will be measured. Common measures are as follows:

Binary (whether or not an event has occurred)   For example, whether or not the subject has experienced a complete or partial response from cancer treatment at 12 months. Typical measures of the event are proportions (risk), rates or odds, and measures of treatment effect include odds ratios and differences in the proportions (or rates) between the intervention and control groups.

Count (the frequency of an event in a set time period)   For example, the number of episodes of epilepsy experienced by patients in a 30-day period. A typical unit of measurement would be the rate (count per unit/time), and measures of treatment effect include incidence density ratios (similar to odds ratios) *or* differences between the rates in the groups being compared.

Time to event (how long it takes to observe the outcome of interest) For example, the survival time of patients with advanced breast cancer. Endpoints of this type usually contain censored data (i.e., the event of interest has not been observed by the end of the follow-up period), and analyses involve comparing "averaged" relative risks or hazard/risk ratios (pooled across the time period of the study) between the groups.

Measurement on a continuous scale   Examples include blood pressure and temperature measurements, and analyses involve comparing the difference between the means of the intervention and control groups.

Other measurements   Included are ordinal scales such as quality-of-life ratings outcomes measured on these scales require specialized statistical methods. Any transformation on data likely to be required before analysis should be discussed. This includes possible groupings or classifications of data (e.g., into good, acceptable and poor quality of life), as well as mathematical transformations (logarithms, square root, etc.) needed to "normalize" the outcome variables. Typically these transformations are used if the distribution of the outcome exhibits distortion, and where, after transformation, this distribution is symmetrical and thus satisfies the assumptions of the statistical method being used to make comparisons.[4] While the underlying assumptions of common statistical tests vary, underpinning all these tests is the assumption that either the outcome (or some transformation of the outcome) or other calculated measures (e.g., correlation coefficients, hazard or odds ratios) will be "normally" distributed. Also reported should be how missing data will be accounted for in the analyses (both scientifically and statistically). For example, missing data are sometimes omitted, assigned the baseline value or the group average, or imputed using statistical theory.[5]

Additionally there should be noted whether statistical inference will be drawn using one-tailed or two-tailed tests (with appropriate justification) and if any statistical adjustments for multiple comparisons will be performed. In reporting the results of randomized trials, an unadjusted analysis for the primary outcome will provide a consistent, unbiased estimate of underlying treatment differences; this is guaranteed by the randomization process. This analysis should usually be the primary comparison. However, if the randomization was stratified, a primary analysis stratified by the stratification factors may be equally appropriate. Subsidiary analyses, which adjust for stratification factors, other potential confounders, or both, can further define the effect of treatment and may provide more efficient statistical comparisons.

Parametric tests are based on specific distributional assumptions such as the normal distribution.[6] Common misconceptions in analyzing clinical data are that a nonparametric analysis (e.g., Wilcoxon rank-sum test) is appropriate if the sample size is small (<30), the data appear skewed (i.e., may not be normally distributed) or that the medians are being compared. Whether the distribution of the data departs significantly from the normal distribution may be formally tested; if no departure from normality is indicated, comparisons based on the normal distribution are usually still preferable. Tests based on the assumption of normally distributed data can also be statistically valid for small sample sizes (as low as three per arm). Of course, if there is clear evidence that the data are not normally distributed, the appropriate statistical tests (e.g., "exact" tests or nonparametric tests) or appropriate data transformations are required. Finally, even nonparametric tests require some assumptions with respect to the underlying populations from which the samples are drawn. If there is a choice of statistical method (i.e., assumptions of a parametric test are satisfied), nonparametric methods are generally not as powerful (i.e., do not have the same ability to detect a significant difference if it actually exists) as their parametric counterparts. A checklist for a statistical analysis plan is provided in the next section.

COMPONENTS OF THE SAP FOR CLINICAL TRIALS

- Provide a detailed description of the primary and secondary endpoints and how they are measured.
- Provide details of the statistical methods and tests that will be used to analyze the endpoints.
- Describe the strategy to be used (e.g., alternative statistical procedures) if the distributional or test assumptions are not satisfied.
- Indicate of whether comparisons will be one-tailed or two-tailed (with appropriate justification if necessary) and specify the level of significance to be used.
- Identify whether any adjustment to the significance level or the final P values will be made to account for any planned or unplanned multiple testing or subgroup analyses.

- Specify potential adjusted analyses with a statement of which covariates or factors will be included.
- Identify any planned subgroup or subset analysis along with justification for the relevance of this analysis (e.g., biological rationale) before commencement of the trial.
- Specify planned exploratory analyses, justifying their importance.
- Support claimed differential subgroup effects with biological rationale as well as evidence from within and outside the study. Provide statistical evidence of interaction between the overall treatment effect and that observed in the subgroup(s) of interest.

Remember, prespecified subgroups will have more interpretive value than those defined on an adhoc basis or as a result of multiple comparisons.

Requirements of the SAP

- The SAP is a clearly defined section within the protocol and approved prior to the start of clinical research study.
- The SAP should include the details of the planned statistical analyses associated with a clinical study. The analyses are planned with the desired work product(s) in mind and should be conducted in a consistent and repeatable manner.
- The SAP should contain the detailed requirements and parameters for the reporting results of the clinical research trial, the format and content of output reports, and the tests to support the robustness and sensitivity of the analysis conducted.
- Recommended checks and specific procedures whose implementation and completion will improve/ensure the quality of the plan and the associated data, as well as prevent study compromise should be included.
- The SAP should include, at a minimum, for each primary and secondary endpoint:

    How the outcome will be measured.

    Any transformations on the data likely to be required before analysis.

    Appropriate statistical tests which will be used to analyze the data.

    How missing data will be accounted for in the analyses (both scientifically and statistically).

Whether statistical inference will be drawn and if any statistical adjustments for multiple comparisons will be performed.

"*P*–Value Isn't Everything"

Suppose that the statistical significance test for the primary endpoint of the study was set at $p \leq 0.05$ and the trial results showed a $p = 0.051$. Does this means that the trial failed because it didn't meet the predetermined significance level? Several factors should be examined before reaching this conclusion:

1. Strength of positive trend toward the pre-set significant level. In this example $p = 0.051$ is a strong trend toward significance.
2. The totality of the data and other supporting endpoints.
3. Safety of the product
4. Marketing advantage issues
   - Simplicity and ease of use
   - Pricing

An example of a study that did not meet the primary endpoint criteria by a slight margin is given in Chapter 3 (HeartMate II study). Although the study did not meet the prespecified success criteria for the primary endpoint, this device was approved by the FDA because the results of this study were not seen to be different from other previous studies. Meeting the primary endpoint in a clinical trial is important, but it is not the only factor considered by the FDA for approval of an investigational device. Some people think that it is really pass–fail: if you miss the primary endpoint, approval is not possible. However, the FDA looks at the totality of the data, the individual components or a composite, as well as the safety issues. At the end of the day, the FDA wants an accurate representation of all the results in the labeling.

ROLES AND RESPONSIBILITIES OF THE CLINICAL PERSONNEL IN COMPLETING THE STUDY PROTOCOL

The roles and responsibilities of the key members of the sponsor's clinical staff in completing clinical studies can be summarized as follows:

Study Statistician

- Ensures that the protocol and any amendments cover all relevant statistical issues clearly and accurately.
- Reviews the CRFs to ensure that primary and secondary endpoints are collected and/or captured appropriately to satisfy analyses called for in the SAP, where applicable.
- Works with the clinical data manager to update the study plan if the SAP changes and if those changes reflect changes to data collected during the conduct of the clinical research trial.

Clinical Study Team

- Conducts the clinical finals and collects outcome data.
- Provides these data to the study statistician on the protocol and SAP.

CHANGING THE PRIMARY OUTCOME DURING THE CONDUCT OF THE STUDY

The primary endpoint is considered the most important outcome because the sample size of the trial is based on this endpoint, is used to assess primary objective of a trial, and is related to the intended use of the therapy. However, sometimes during the course of a trial new information is generated and leads to changes to endpoints. This new information may include, for example, results from other trials or identification of better biomarkers or surrogate outcome measures. Such changes can allow incorporation of up-to-date knowledge into the trial design. The following questions should be asked when considering changing the endpoints after the initiation of the study: What is the source of the new information that triggers consideration of a change in endpoints? Have interim data on the endpoint (or related data) been reviewed? Who is making the decision to change endpoints? Are trial sponsors involved, or is there an independent external advisory committee?

The important consideration when evaluating whether to modify an endpoint is whether the decision is independent of the data obtained from the trial. If the decision to revise endpoints is independent of the data from the trial, then such revisions may have merit. Some trials have successfully changed endpoints after the trials began by maintaining independence between the decision and the trial data.[7,8] If, however, the decision to change an endpoint is not independent of the trial data, then there is a serious concern because any new endpoints may display a trend toward significance while any discarded candidate endpoints may fail to display the desirable trend.

To evaluate whether a change in endpoint is independent of data analysis from the trial, investigators and reviewers should ask three questions. First, what is the source of the new information that leads to the change in endpoints? If the source is external to the trial in question, for example, arising from results from another trial, then the revision of endpoints may be credible. Second, have interim data on the endpoint (or related data) from a trial been reviewed or subjected to interim analysis? If the trial data have not been reviewed, then the revision of endpoints may again be necessary. Third, who is making the decision regarding endpoint revision (e.g., trial sponsors or an independent external advisory committee)? It is important that decision makers not to have knowledge of the endpoint (or related trial data) results. So study sponsors, investigators, and the Data Monitoring Safety Board may not be appropriate decision makers for endpoint revisions.

The changes to the endpoint should be documented in the amended protocol, and revised SAP. A clear statement should be given in the amended protocol describing the changes to endpoints, the information obtained after the start of the trial that led to these changes, the reasons for these changes, and the decision-making procedure. The reasons given should explain why the endpoints were excluded from the analyses and whether this decision was independent of the trial data.

Secondary Outcomes

Analysis of the secondary outcomes needs to be conducted in the same as for the primary outcome, with sufficient documentation in the analysis plan as to how the results will be implemented. Need for further exploratory analyses should be identified where indicated before the completion of the study, with a clear scientific rationale provided for value of such additional analyses.

Description of Study Endpoints

Study endpoints are regarded as "hard" or "soft" endpoints. The characteristics of these endpoints follow: Not all endpoints can be classified. Some endpoints are useful and reliable but require some subjectivity. Examples of these endpoints are pathology endpoints. In principle, the endpoint should be chosen based on clinical relevance and on the sample size of the study, which should have a sufficient power to detect a clinically meaningful difference.

"Hard" Endpoints

- "Hard" endpoints are quantitative measurements. These endpoints must be:
    - Well-defined in study protocol
    - Definitive with respect to disease process
    - Not subjective
- Examples are death, time to disease progression/relapse, and some laboratory measurement.

Soft Endpoints   Soft endpoints are not directly related to disease process. So soft endpoints do not require subjective assessments by patient/physician. Examples are Quality of Life and Symptom questionnaires.

DEFINITION OF PRIMARY AND SECONDARY ENDPOINTS

A primary endpoint is defined as "a clinical endpoint that provides sufficient evidence to fully categorize clinically the effect of a treatment that would support a regulatory claim for the treatment." A secondary endpoint is defined as "an additional clinical characterization of a treatment that could not alone be convincing of a clinically significant treatment effect."

COMBINED "COMPOSITE" ENDPOINTS

A combined endpoint is an endpoint that could present several complications such as death, myocardial infarction (MI), or revascularization. The procedure to use when a combined endpoint is a probability is as follows:

- Decrease sample size.
- Ensure that trials are clinically meaningful, and biologically related (nonfatal myocardial infarction and cardiac death).

- Create a hierarchy of potential problems by pathologic risk:

    Death > MI > revascularization

    Rare versus common event

    Biologic pathway? If not the same, components may go in opposite directions!

- Follow up time and censoring information for each participant. The method of analysis is often event-time exposition.

SURROGATE ENDPOINTS

Surrogate endpoints reflect the clinical outcome of the investigational therapy (surrogate marker, or intermediate endpoint) as are:

- Used when definitive endpoint trial would be too long or costly. Surrogate endpoint trial generally smaller because there are involved:

    Continuous measurements

    More frequent events

- Generally accepted if:

    Measurements appear to be accurate and reliable

    Acceptable to the participants (invasive?) and investigators (cost, ease of use?)

Examples of Surrogate Endpoints

Examples of the use of surrogate endpoints in clinical studies are listed in Table 1.1.

TABLE 1.1   Example of Surrogate Endpoints

Disease	Definitive Endpoints	Surrogate Endpoints
Cardiovascular disease	Myocardial infarction	Cholesterol level
	Heart failure	BNP
	Stroke	Blood pressure
Cancer	Mortality	Tumor size reduction
Prostate cancer	Disease progression	PSA
HIV infection	AIDS/death	CD4 + count
Glaucoma	Vision loss	Intraocular pressure

Problems with Surrogate Endpoints

The effect of encainide and flecainide on mortality in a randomized trial of arrhythmia suppression after myocardial infarction has been studied in the Cardiac Arrhythmia Suppression Trial (CAST).[9] The occurrence of ventricular premature depolarization in survivors of myocardial infarction is a risk factor for subsequent sudden death, but whether anti-arrhythmic therapy reduces the risk is not known. In this trial suppression of asymptomatic ventricular arrhythmia was hypothesized to be surrogate for arrhythmatic death, but the surrogate and mortality endpoints had conflicting results. The CAST study evaluated the effects of anti-arrhythmic therapy (encainide, flecainide, or moricizine) in patients with asymptomatic or mildly symptomatic ventricular arrhythmia of the 2309 patients recruited, 1727 (75%) had initial suppression of their arrhythmia (as assessed by Holter recording) through the use of one of the three study drugs and had been randomly assigned to receive an active drug or a placebo. Over an average of 10 months of follow-up, the patients treated with the active drug had a higher rate of death from arrhythmia than the patients assigned to the placebo. They also accounted for the higher total mortality rate, 56 of 730 (7.7%), and 22 of 725 (3.0%), respectively; relative risk, 2.5; 95% confidence interval, 1.6 to 4.5. The study concluded that neither encainide nor flecainide should be used in the treatment of patients with asymptomatic or minimally symptomatic ventricular arrhythmia after myocardial infarction, even though these drugs may be effective initially in suppressing ventricular arrhythmia.

Criteria for a "Good" Surrogate Endpoint   The following factors contribute to the selection of good surrogate endpoints:

- Change in surrogate is strongly correlated with change in clinical outcome.
- Surrogate is in the biological pathway of the disease.
- There is strong statistical association.
- Latency time is short (↑ surrogate followed by rapid onset of disease).
- Patient is responsive to treatment (but: effect on disease often not predicted by effect on surrogate).

Sample Size Determination of a Clinical Study   Sample size calculations depend on the following parameters:

- Type I error rate (α), which is normally set up at 0.05.
- Type II error rate ($1 - \beta$), which is usually set up at least 80%.
- Endpoint to be analyzed.
- Statistical method to be used in analyzing the endpoint.
- Estimated value for the endpoint one expects to see in the control arm.
- Estimated improvement one expects to see in the treatment arm (clinical outcome benefit, e.g., reduction of mortality by 10%).
- Amount of variation in the endpoint measured.

Endpoint to Be Analyzed

Endpoint measurement can take one of the following forms:

- Yes/no responses
- Continuous responses
- Questionnaire data
- Survival from event following a long period of time
- Repeated measures of an outcome over several weeks

REDUCING THE STUDY'S SAMPLE SIZE

The sample size of the study can be decreased by manipulating the following parameters:

- Allowing for a bigger type I error.
- Allowing for a bigger type II error.
- Increasing the level of improvement one expects to achieve.
- Choosing a more powerful way of testing.
- For a binary endpoint, choosing the one that is closest to 50% in likelihood of being observed in the control arm.
- For survival endpoints, extending the length of follow-up.
- For continuous measures, decreasing the variation in the outcome.

STATISTICAL TERMS TO DEFINE ENDPOINT MEASUREMENTS

The following statistical parameters are used to estimate the results of interest:

- Percentage of patients with the event
- Mean of the outcome
- Kaplan–Meier rate of survival
- Ratio of percentages
- Differences in percentages

The following statistic terms are used in clinical research:

Mean   The average across a group of patients.

Median   The 50th percentile. This is the value such that half the group falls below it and half the group is above it.

Variance   A measure of how far the data fall from the mean. To calculate variance, take each patient's data and subtract it from the mean. Square the difference to get rid of the negative signs. Add up all of these squared deviations and divide the total by N (the number of patients) to obtain the average squared deviation.

Standard deviation   The square root of the variance. Variance is on a squared scale. Taking the square root puts it back on the same scale as the original values.

p-Value   This is a probability value. It is the probability of obtaining the existing results or even more extreme results if the effect observed is really due to random chance alone.

The study protocol should include:

- The hypothesis (or hypotheses) that is to be tested by the study
- The test that will be used on the hypothesis
- The critical value for declaring significance (type I error rate)
- For the primary hypothesis, we usually use a critical value of 0.05.
- According to this rule, if we complete the study and the p-values are close to 0.05 (on either side), then we consider these p-values to be "borderline" in significance or we could say that there is a "trend" toward a significant difference.
- The further a p-value is from 0.05, the more we can believe that it is a true effect (when smaller than 0.05) or that there is no true difference in the groups (when larger than 0.05).

Confidence intervals   Definition of a 95% confidence interval (CI):

If you were to do the study an infinite number of times, then 95% of the estimates of effect would fall within the bounds of the interval.

Relationship between *p*-Values and CI

1. Decide how you want to look at the treatment effect (the point estimate).

   Difference:

$$15.7 - 14.2 = \text{change of 1.5 in death/MI rates}$$

   Percent change:

$$1.5/15.7 = 9.5\% \text{ decrease in rates}$$

   Odds ratio (O.R.):

   0.89 odds of death/MI for Integrilin compared with a placebo

2. Test that treatment effect and calculate the *p*-value.

   $p = 0.042$, that the O.R. of 0.89 is different than an O.R. of 1.0, or that the difference in rates of 1.5% is significantly greater than 0.

3. Calculate the 95% CI to determine how robust that effective size is.

   CI of $(0.794, 0.996)$ does not include 1 but is very close.

   The *p*-value and 95% confidence interval are calculated from the data using exactly the same measures.

   Usually the same measure of effective size is used and the same measure of how much variation existed in the outcome in the study.

   Each *p*-value indicates the chance that a result is attributable to a random occurrence alone.

   p-Values each show how likely the results seen are due to random occurrences.

   If the confidence interval contains the value for no difference (O.R. = 1, difference = 0), then it is estimated that there is more than a 5% chance that any differences noted were random occurrence. If not, then there is less than a 5% chance of occurrence.

If one of the bounds is the value for no difference, then there is about a 5% chance that the results were random occurrences.

The width of the confidence interval also is an indication of the range of values that the true effect size likely falls within.

Interpreting the Significance of the Results

- Is the effect size clinically meaningful?
- Is the sample very homogeneous—to whom are the results generalized?
- How close is the p-value to 0.05?
- Does the confidence interval include the estimate of no difference (1 for O.R., 0 for differences, or % change)?
- How wide are the confidence intervals?

REPORTING RESULTS OF CLINICAL TRIALS

The following are recommendations to avoid common mistakes in reporting the results of a clinical trial.

Reporting Scale

- Spell out acronym.
- Define measure description.
- Indicate the range of direction of the score (e.g., 0 is the best, and 10 is the worst).

Defining Category

- Provide category title.
- If category is based on continuous measures, determine the threshold when is possible.
- Report possible outcomes (e.g., improved and not improved).
- Provide time period of assessment.
- Provide information on how was the improvement or no improvement determined.

Outcome Tables

- Define rows (measures or counts) and columns (arms or comparison groups) to be logically consistent.
- Provide cell (data) measures or counts derived from participants within arms or groups:
    Measure type (and measure of dispersion) needs to be consistent with data being reported.
    Unit of measure must be consistent with values.
- Give absolute values and percentages (absolute values are preferable to percentages).

Precision of Outcome Measure Information

- Outcome measure title, and description headings, should include:
    Name and description of measure so that it is informative to people not familiar with study
    If categorized, description of categories
- Units should directly reflect data in the table.
- Viewers of the table should be able to understand what the numbers represent.

Reporting of Adverse Events

- Report using two different tables for "serious" and "other" (nonserious) adverse events.
    Do not report any serious adverse events in the "other" adverse events table.
    If possible, indicate the level of severity to distinguish "serious" from "other" adverse events (e.g., mild, moderate, and severe) in the "other" table.
- If no adverse events occurred, enter 0 for the "total number affected" data items.
- Distinguish between procedure and procedure-related adverse events. In some surgical trials all adverse events occurring within 30 days of the procedure are regarded as procedure-related adverse events
- Distinguish between device-related and unrelated adverse events. If an adverse event is designated as a device related, then

a causality relationship between the adverse event and investigational product should be established.

SUPERIORITY AND EQUIVALENCE TRIALS

Superiority versus Noninferiority Trials

Superiority Design   Show that the new treatment is better than the control or standard treatment.

Noninferiority   Show that the new treatment:

1. Is not worse that the standard by more than some margin.
2. Would have surpassed the placebo if a placebo arm had been included (regulatory).

Noninferiority Trial

- Question whether new (easier or cheaper) treatment is as good as the current treatment.
- Specify margin of "equivalence" or noninferiority.
- Because equivalency cannot be statistically proved, show that the difference is less than something with specified probability.
- Provide historical evidence of patients' sensitivity to treatment.
- If the sample size was small, which leads to low power and subsequently lack of significant difference, do not imply "equivalence."

Optimaal Trial

For the OPTIMAAL trial[10] (OPtimal Trial In Myocardial Infarction with the Angiotensin II Antagonist Losartan), the rationale was as follows:

- ACE inhibitors reduce mortality in high-risk post-MI patients.
- Selective Angiotensin II receptor antagonists are an alternative because they more completely block the tissue Renin-Angiotensin system (RAS).
- A better tolerability hypothesis was the basis for the study.
- The question was wether losartan (50 mg) is superior or noninferior to captopril (150 mg) in decreasing all-cause mortality in high-risk patients following the AMI study design.

- The study was designed as double-blind, randomized, parallel, investigator-initiated, no placebo control.
- Event-driven study outcome was all-cause death (937); 499 in the losartan group, and 447 in the captopril arm.
- A total of 5477 patients were involved in the multicenter study, located in Denmark, Finland, Germany, Ireland, Norway, Sweden, and the United Kingdom.
- Captopril was the comparator.
- Captopril has well-documented benefits.
- Captopril at 50 mg 3 times daily has an indication for CHF worldwide.
- Captopril is widely used, and available as a generic drug.

Study Results The Angiotensin II antagonist losartan failed to show benefit over the ACE inhibitor captopril in this trial. Captopril showed trend towards superiority with regard to the primary endpoint—all-cause mortality. Reported was that a total of 937 deaths, 447 in the captopril (16.2%), and 499 (18.2%) in the losartan arm, with a *p*-value of 0.069 and 95% CI of 1.13 (0.99 – 1.28). However, losartan showed significantly better tolerability than captopril.

Hypothesis

Losartan (50 mg) is superior or noninferior to captopril (150 mg) in decreasing all-cause mortality in high-risk patients following anterior myocardial infarction (AMI).

Study Design

- Double-blind, randomized, parallel, investigator-initiated, no placebo control
- Event driven (all-cause death = 937)
- Multicenter (Denmark, Finland, Germany, Ireland, Norway, Sweden, United Kingdom)

Captopril as Comparator

- Captopril has well-documented benefits.
- Captopril at 50 mg 3 times daily has an indication for CHF worldwide.

- Captopril is widely used, and available as a generic drug.
- Required for 95% power were 937 deaths to detect a 20% difference between groups.
- A noninferiority margin of 10% was chosen based on placebo-controlled trials of ACE-inhibitors.
- Analysis was by intention-to-treat and the Cox regression model.

Assay Sensitivity

- Ability to distinguish an effective treatment from a less effective or ineffective treatment.
- Different implications of lack of assay sensitivity:

    Superiority trials that fail to show the test treatment to be superior thus fail to lead to a conclusion of efficacy.

- Noninferiority trials that show an ineffective treatment to be noninferior thus lead to an erroneous conclusion of efficacy.

Superiority trials test for statistically significant and clinically meaningful improvements (or harm!) from the use of the experimental treatment over the results obtained through the use of standard care.

Noninferiority Study Design: selecting the noninferiority Margin[11,12]

1. Set the noninferiority margin (M) to half the point of estimate Δ.
2. FDA proposes that M to be set to half the lower limit of CI for Δ from meta-analysis of previous studies.
3. Clinical judgment is based on the difference in event rates that makes the two treatments no longer "therapeutically equivalent." Because therapeutic equivalence is not well defined, companies must meet with the FDA in advance to agree on noninferiority margin.

Example for Selecting Noninferiority Margin In the TARGET4 trial,[13] two glycoprotein IIa/IIIb inhibitors, tirofiban and abciximab, were studied to establish the noninferiority of tirofiban in prevention of cardiovascular events in patients undergoing PCI. The primary endpoint was death, MI, or urgent revascularization in 30 days. The noninferiority margin for the hazard ratio was chosen as 1.47, half the effect of abciximab in the EPISTENT trial. The estimated hazard ratio and its 95% confidence interval were 1.26 (1.01, 1.57). The investigators concluded that T was inferior to A. The trial design was criticized because an agent that increased the event rate by 47% would not have been considered to be therapeutically equivalent to abciximab.

Similarly, in the SPORTIF trials 5,[14] ximelegatran was compared to warfarin for stroke prevention in patients with atrial fibrillation. Again, based on the historical evidence, the sponsor chose an absolute non-inferiority margin of 2%. The event rates in the warfarin group (control) were 2.3% (Sportif III) and 1.2% (Sportif V). Because of the low event rates in the control arm, the noninferiority margin allowed the conclusion of noninferiority, even with a doubling of the event rate in the ximelegatran arm.

The common theme in these trials was that a noninferiority margin based on the effect of the comparator drug was not consistent with the community standard for therapeutic equivalence. In response to these and other trials, the FDA began to take a more conservative stance about the choice of the noninferiority margin. This caused FDA statisticians to advocate the 95–95, or the two confidence interval, method. In this method, M is set equal to the lower 95% confidence limit for Δ based on the data from the historical placebo controlled trials. In the noninferiority trial, the upper confidence limit for the effect of T relative to C must be less than this value. That is, the CI for Δ from the historical data and the CI for $pT–pC$ must not overlap. This criterion is sometimes impossibly stringent and depends directly on the strength of the evidence in the historical trials.

In the PRoFess trial 6,[15] the investigators sought to demonstrate the noninferiority of aspirin plus dipyridamole relative to an active control, clopidogrel, for the prevention of recurrent stroke. Following the 95–95 approach, they chose a noninferiority margin equal to half the lower limit of the confidence interval from placebo-controlled trials of clopidogrel. This gave a noninferiority margin for the hazard ratio of 1.075. To achieve a manageable sample size, the investigators chose an alternative hypothesis that T would reduce the event rate by 6.5%, that is, that A + D would actually be superior to clopidogrel. In the trial the observed event rates were almost identical [9.0% (A + D) and 8.8% (C), RR = 1.01 (0.92, 1.11)], but the data did not satisfy the prespecified noninferiority criterion.

SUBGROUP ANALYSIS

Subgroup analysis is addressed in greater detail in Chapter 2. Potential subgroup analyses should be specified before the commencement of a study to guard against data "dredging" or "trawling." Applying many different statistical tests to the same data (e.g., on subgroups or different outcomes) has the effect of greatly increasing the chance that at least one of these comparisons will be declared statistically significant even if there is no real difference. This practice is often termed data dredging. However, simply specifying a subgroup analysis in advance does not necessarily add scientific legitimacy to the interpretation. A number of strategies exist to ensure the credibility of subgroup analyses, that there is a biological rationale for considering the subgroup separately from the rest of the patients in the study. Lack of strong biological or clinical evidence for why the treatment should have different effects in a particular subgroup would detract from support of a true underlying differential effect, even if a conventionally significant difference were found. That there is prior evidence or belief that a differential treatment effect in a subgroup is plausible. Lack of prior evidence suggests that differential treatment effects observed in subgroups become hypothesis-generating observations rather than firm conclusions, that there is statistical evidence (i.e., a significant interaction) of a difference in the effect of treatment for the subgroup in question compared with the other patients. For example, if there is an apparent advantage of treatment in younger compared with older patients, then careful (clinical and statistical) examination of this difference is required before it can be confidently concluded that a true differential treatment benefit exists in the subgroup of younger patients. Studies are frequently underpowered to detect such interaction effects; nevertheless, lack of statistical evidence of such interaction should prohibit firmly concluding any differential treatment effect in the subgroup, that there is independent confirmation from other factors in the study of the possible differential treatment effect in the subgroup. For example, if, in a trial examining the effect of chemotherapy in gastric cancer, it is observed that women survive longer after an intervention than men, supporting evidence could be to observe that the response rate to treatment was higher and time to disease progression was also longer in women compared with men. Common pitfalls with subgroup analysis are focusing on the size of the p-value and of the treatment effect in any subgroup, ignoring the play of chance. Other factors, such as the total number of subgroups examined, also play a major role in determining the credibility of an observed differential subgroup effect. Subgroups defined before initiating the study would be more credible in terms of true differences in effect on the study findings than those determined only at the time of analysis.

Logistics of Subgroup Analysis

When the overall result fails to show efficacy, usually subgroup findings are not acceptable and subgroup analyses at best can be exploratory or hypothesis-generating analyses. When one starts to do multiple subgroup testing, one can easily make a false positive claim based on such subgroup analysis. We do not know how to interpret the *p*-values based on such post hoc analysis. Furthermore, without replication of the results in a second well-controlled study, the subgroup analysis cannot be ruled out for a false positive result. The sponsor wished to claim approval based on a subgroup of patients, however, and this subgroup hypothesis was not stated as a hypothesis of interest to be tested in the original protocol. All subgroup hypotheses need to be stated in the protocol, and accordingly the proper allocation of α has to be specified. Otherwise, such post hoc subgroup claim will inflate the type I error, making it difficult to interpret these *p*-values.

CHALLENGES TO ICF

The conduct of clinical trials is founded on the protection of human rights and the dignity of the human being (the Helsinki Declaration). The guiding principles of informed consent are as follows:

- Nuremberg Code
    Subjects must give voluntary consent.
    Subjects are free to drop out of clinical trials.
- The Belmont Report: Respect for Persons
    Subjects are autonomous agents and should be treated with respect.
    Informed consent must be freely and voluntarily given.
    Subjects of diminished capacity require additional protections.

Code of Federal Regulations Protecting Human Subjects

- DHHS: 45 CFR Part 46—Subpart A: Protection of Human Subjects
- FDA: 21 CFR Part 50
- Additional DHHS Regulations 45 CFR 46-Subpart B: Pregnant Women, Human Fetuses, and Neonates in Research (in 2001)

Subpart C: Biomedical and Behavioral Research Involving Prisoners as Subjects (in 1978)

Subpart D: Children Involved as Subjects in Research (in 1983)

Informed Consent Process

Three key components, subsequent to the Belmont Report, are that the subject:

1. Receive full information
2. Demonstrate complete understanding
3. Voluntarily agree to participate

Basic Elements of the ICF

The ICF contains the following elements of the protocol:

1. Title of the protocol
2. Number of subjects to be enrolled
3. Identity of the sponsor
4. Invitation to participate
5. Purpose, duration, and procedures
6. Foreseeable risks
7. Expected benefits
8. Alternative treatments
9. Confidentiality conditions
10. Compensation for injury
11. Contact persons for questions on both research care related questions and human subjects' protection questions
12. Voluntary nature of participation
13. Circumstances under which subjects participation may be terminated
14. Consequences of discontinuing research participation
15. How notification of significant new findings will be explained
16. Anticipated costs
17. Identifying the person(s) who will review the subjects' records

Conditions for Waiver of Required Elements

A waiver for ICF could be obtained based on the following elements:

1. Minimal risk
2. No adverse effects on the rights and welfare of the subjects
3. Trial cannot not be practicably carried out without the waiver
4. Subjects provided with additional information after participation

Challenges of Writing an Informed Consent Document

Readability   Because of poor literacy skills in the United States, it is recommended that for easy readability the ICF:

- Be easily understandable
- Be written at the eighth-grade reading level
- Have all technical terms defined
- Give explicit information
- Give concrete examples
- Highlight critical terms
- Give clear purpose of the study
- Discuss prior knowledge and information
- Use mental images

Comprehension   The following tips are recommended to enhance the comprehension of the ICF:

- Shorten words by removing unnecessary prefixes and suffixes, using simple synonyms.
- Remember that average readable sentence length in American English is 17 words long.
- Sentences are considered too long if they contain more than 30 words.
- If you read a sentence out loud and have to pause for a breath, the sentence needs punctuation or is too long!
- Organize a visual presentation:
    Arrange contents under topical headings or short questions.
    Use the active voice and personalize the document to the patient.
    Use a font size is at least 12 points.
    Be aware that the quality of print and paper affects readability.
    Appropriatly use illustrations to improve comprehension.

Signatures on the ICF Document

By signing the informed consent document, the subject/participant or legally authorized representative (LAR) is indicating his/her willingness to participate after receiving information about the study. Additional signatures may be required (e.g., PI, witness).

Who Can Obtain the Consent?

The principle investigator (PI) or associate investigator (AI) can obtain consent assuming that this person will have the following. Peroons other than the PI or AI must be approved by IRB.

- Knowledgeable about the informed consent process.
- Knowledgeable about the study's protocol.
- Means to determine that the subject is well informed and is making a free and uncoerced decision.
- Means to identify and resolve outstanding questions.

When Will Consent Be Obtained?

Subject consent must be obtained prior to any procedures (screening consent), after protocol eligibility criteria are met (treatment protocol consent), and after sufficient time is allowed for subjects to discuss what the Investigator said about the protocol with family, friends, and other physicians.

How Will Consent Be Obtained?

The best way to obtain the subject's consent is usually by:

- Discussion style with questions and answers
- Allowing the potential subject time to review the treatment protocol prior to consent
- Use of additional aids
- Use of written consent form approved by IRB
- Voluntary consent, without undue coercion

After the signature is obtained, the original signed document is filed in the subject's medical record and a copy of the consent is given to the patient.

"Short Form" Consent Process

The person obtaining consent must have:

1. Witness/Interpreter present during the consenting process/discussion and Q&A.
   a. Witness must be fluent in English and the language of the subject.
   b. Witness may serve as the interpreter.
   c. Witness can not be a family member or close personal friend of the subject (to help avoid coercion from the family and miscommunication of the consent process).
2. An English version of the current IRB approved consent form.
3. A "short-form," IRB approved consent translated into the subject's language.
4. All material outlined in the IRB approved consent presented orally to the interpreter who will then convey the information to the subject.
   a. Interpreter does not have to be read the consent word for word.
   b. Interpreter may present the information directly to the subject if he/she speaks the same language as the subject.

Ethical Considerations in the Informed Consent Process

The following issues should be carefully addressed when designing or executing the ICF:

- How to understand and measure someone's capacity to consent?
- How to protect those with limited capacity?
- How much information should be and how is best presented?
- How to assure subject's understanding?
- What is voluntary?
- How to avoid undue influence?
- What are acceptable ways of demonstrating consent?

Documentation of Informed Consent Process

Specific to in the patient's medical record should be a statement indicating:

- Protocol name and number
- Version of consent form signed
- That all questions were reviewed and answered
- Who obtained the actual signature
- Individuals present during consent
- Verification that a copy was given to the patient

Re-consenting Study Subject

New findings (toxicities) may require re-consent from the study subject:

- The investigator is required to inform subject of new findings and to ensure that they are still willing to participate on clinical trial.
- The willingness of subject to continue must be documented in the medical record.
- The subject may be required by the IRB, or sponsor, to sign the IRB approved updated consent form.

Consenting Vulnerable Subjects

When consenting vulnerable subjects, the following situation should be carefully addressed. Children who turn 18 years old are required to sign an IRB approved updated consent form.

- Assent is the child's affirmative agreement to participate in research.
- Failure of subject to object should not be construed as assent.
- IRBs may waive the requirement for assent (capacity-based waiver).
- Children have insufficient capacity to participate in the decision.
- Direct benefit to the child must be demonstrated.
- IRB determines if a separate assent document is required as opposed to verbal consent/agreement of the child.
- A child's verbal assent needs to be indicated on the consent document.
- Age appropriateness needs to be considered.
- The maturity level of the child must be considered.
- The psychological state due to the disease is also a factor.

- Level of comprehension and reasoning can be altered by:
    Anxiety
    Physical disturbances
    Emotional disturbances

Signatures on the Consent Documents

"Short forms" 21 CFR 50.27 and 46 CFR 46.117 are IRB approved. These forms should be:

- Signed by subject
- Signed by witness/translator
- Signed by investigator
- Signed by witness/translator

ICF Requirement Exceptions

Exceptions from ICF requirements may include the following situations:

- A life threatening situation necessitating the use of a test article.
- Subject's inability to communicate consent, or to give legally effective consent.
- In sufficient time to obtain consent from the subject's legal representative.
- No alternative method of approval or generally recognized therapy available that provides an equal or greater like hood of saving the subject's life.

Exception from ICF for Planned Emergency Research[16,17]

In planned emergency research where the subject is unable to provide consent, the ICF can be waived by the FDA in this situation.

RISK/BENEFIT ANALYSIS

Every medical research project involving human subjects should be preceded by careful assessment of predictable risks and burdens in comparison with foreseeable benefits to the subject or to others. This does not preclude the participation of healthy volunteers in medical research. (Helsinki Declaration)

All bioethics principles, as derived from the Nuremberg Code, the Helsinki Declaration, and the Belmont Report, require that human research be initiated if the anticipated benefit(s) for the research subject and society outweigh the risks. The risk/benefit ratio of a clinical study should be determined by the sponsor, investigator, IRB, and the reviewing regulatory body. This section in the protocol or investigational plan contains the following analyses:

1. Risks due to disease or condition
2. Risks associated with alternative treatments
3. Risks associated with the investigational product
4. Potential benefits of the investigational product
5. Risk/benefit assessment of the investigational product

There is a major challenge to certain clinical studies that have not shown a direct benefit to the individual study subject, usually a healthy volunteer for drug (e.g., phase I studies) and medical device clinical trials (e.g., diagnostic devices). To justify the conduct of these studies, a clear benefit(s) to society has to be demonstrated.

Challenges to Managing the Study

Clinical trials constitute the single most expensive component of medical device or drug research and development. A cost-effective clinical trial management system yields immediate cost savings for clinical operations and clearance of the product by the regulatory agencies.

This chapter considers compliance issues related to management of study data generated that will be incorporated in the study clinical report. The issues include:

The Design and Management of Medical Device Clinical Trials: Strategies and Challenges, by Salah Abdel-aleem
Copyright © 2010 John Wiley & Sons, Inc.

- Impact of protocol deviations and missing data on study's outcome
- Treatment analyses: intent to treat per protocol
- Subgroup analysis
- Data integrity and quality assurance measures
- Adverse event definition and reporting

The following sets of recommendations are put forward to meet the challenges associated with these issues:

- Instructions and recommendations on how to deal with protocol deviations and missing data in clinical trials
- Mitigation of the negative impact of missing data analysis on the outcome of the study
- Advantages and limitations of the use of certain study analyses, such as the intention-to-treat analysis (which may include the entire study population) and protocol deviations (missed follow-up visits, etc.)
- Subgroup analyses involving multiple testings, the statistical power of a particular subgroup, and the subgroup analyses planned before commencement of the study
- Data integrity and use of quality measurements that protect the quality of data
- Adverse event reporting, including detailed descriptions, time periods required for reporting, and organizations to which adverse events are reported

This chapter provides essential information for study monitors, clinical research associates (CRAs), project managers, and study coordinators at biotechnology and pharmaceutical companies, contract research organizations, and investigational sites on how to manage trials effectively and resolve the challenging issues. The data management section of this chapter details the processes of collecting, entering, reviewing, and cleaning up study data. It also provides guidance on data management plan development. The biostatistics and results interpretation section discusses the role and importance of biostatistics in designing and conducting scientifically sound clinical trials. It also covers the interpretation of trial data. The data management issues, however, are discussed from the clinical trial operational point of view, without detailed statistical analyses. Detailed statistical analyses are behind the scope of this book.

ENHANCING PATIENT ENROLLMENT BY RELAXATION OF STUDY CRITERIA[18,19]

Enhancing subject enrollment is one of the basic requirements of clinical trials, particularly if enrollment is proceeding at a slow rate. There are two ways to enhance enrollment in clinical studies.

Deleting One or More Inclusion/Exclusion Criteria

Provided that a revision of study criteria will not compromise patient safety, stability, patient population, or study endpoints, such modification may include revising the age requirement for the study, or deleting a particular prognostic baseline factor. For example, the participants' age range in clinical studies could be extended to include 80-year-old or older subjects, unless there is a particular reason to select a study-specific patient age group. However, it should be noted that clinical trials that open enrollment to patients older than 85 years old are usually associated with increased adverse events. Adverse event may then not be due to the investigational product but to the aged group. Still some clinical trials open patient enrollment to age ranging from 18 to 65 years old, and this criterion can be relaxed to include even older patients unless the safety, patient population, or study endpoint will be compromised.

In cardiogenic shock trials, for example, where patient enrollment usually proceeds at very slow rate because of the unavailability of patients, a trial may be further compromised by criteria that excludes patients with diabetes. Patients with diabetes roughly constitute 25% of cardiogenic shock patients, so excluding diabetic patients can amount to the reduction of an available pool of patients by 25%. As mentioned above, this restriction could be lifted as long as the change does not affect the safety, patient population, or study endpoints.

Deleting a Protocol/Restricting Procedural Step

The use of a certain medication may be a protocol restricting step, particularly if there is no justification for the medication. Some clinical trials require a medication to be administered for long periods of time or indefinitely. An example is anticoagulant medications taken with the drug-eluting stents. In the United States physicians tend to use certain anticoagulants, such as Plavix, whereas in the EU countries an anticoagulant such as aspirin may be used for economic reasons. So, when designing a global clinical trial that includes international sites, it is recommended that to enhance patient enrollment at these sites, alternatives to Plavix be considered if this does not compromise the safety of the subjects.

In summary, the recommendation for relaxing study criteria to enhance subject enrollment is that relaxation of one or more study criteria may be considered provided that patient safety, stability, patient population structure, and study endpoints are not compromised.

COMPLIANCE WITH THE STUDY PROTOCOL

Research using human subjects should be performed in compliance with the approved clinical protocol to ensure their rights and well-being, as well as the quality and integrity of the safety and efficacy data. These objectives are met by:

1. Selecting study subjects in accordance to the inclusion/exclusion criteria in the study protocol.
2. Following the protocol procedure for treating the subjects.
3. Accurately recording the safety and efficacy data in the study.
4. Accurately documenting and reporting adverse events, serious adverse events, and unanticipated adverse events in the study.
5. Reporting protocol deviations and violations.

To ensure the compliance with the study protocol, investigators should sign a document indicating their adherence to the approved clinical protocol. The investigators and research staff should attend the initiation visit training conducted prior to the start of subject enrollment in the study. This visit is designed to train the investigator and research staff about the investigational device, the clinical protocol procedures, and the principals of GCP.

Implementations of Protocol Compliance

Protocol compliance is incumbent on:

1. The site investigator and research staff who conduct the trial.
2. The sponsor who appoints monitors or representatives to ensure compliance.
3. IRB/EC written procedures and review of the trial.
4. FDA and other regulatory personnel who review and inspect the study.

TABLE 2.1 Criteria for Reproducible Clinical Research

Research Component	Requirement
Data	Availability of the analytical data set
Documentation	Adequate documentation of available data set, electronic files, software information, and programs used to analyze data
Methods	Methods used to access the software, data, coding underlying figures, and tables

Raw Data and Analyzed Data

Data items considered to be raw data are defined as:

- CT scan
- Pulmonary function test
- Death certificate
- Medical record

Data items considered to be analyzed data are:

- "Processed" numerical data presented in graphs and tables.
- Decisions made during an analysis.
- Complex statistical models often containing summarized data.
- Assessed sensitivity of results to key model assumptions.

Criteria for reproducible clinical research are defined in Table 2.1.

CHALLENGES ASSOCIATED WITH DATA ACCURACY AND COMPLETENESS

Potential areas of inaccurate or incomplete data in clinical studies include:

- CRFs: Incomplete write-over corrections in clinical research findings.
- Reporting of adverse events: Missing information about inadequacies occurring in the study.
- Protocol deviations: Inclusion/exclusion criteria deviations, or serious protocol compliance deviations.

A data audit by the FDA may lead to a bioresearch monitoring program (BIMO) inspection. The negative consequences that can result are:

- Holdup of marketing application approval
- FDA refusal to consider suspect data or data for the study
- FDA issuing the 483 warning letter
    These letters are directed to the study sponsor and/or clinical investigator
    Information in the letter is publicly available

Integrity Hold

If the FDA has concerns about the integrity of data, it can place the company on "integrity hold." The company then must:

- Stop the study or studies.
- Submit to a third-party clinical systems audit (similar to BIMO audit).
- Validate/verify all data points for all patients enrolled in the study or studies.
- Submit a corrective action plan (CAP) to the FDA.
- Submit to a second BIMO inspection to ensure that the CAP has been adequately implemented.
- Obtain third-party data certification for subsequent submissions.
- Obtain validation that the data submitted is accurate.

Application Integrity Policy (AIP)

- FDA stops review of applications.
- No new applications will be accepted for review.
- List of firms for which FDA has invoked AIP is publicly available.
- AIP must be formally revoked.
    Audits
    Corrective action plan
    Withdrawal of submissions
- Other FDA investigations may follow by:
  - Office of Criminal Investigation (OCI)
  - Additional investigation from CDRH

Study Source Documents

The following are examples of source documents used in clinical studies:

1. Source data: All information in original records, original records of clinical findings, observations.
2. Source documents: Original data and records (hospital records, office charts, laboratory notes, subjects' evaluation notes, pharmacy records, recorded data from automated instruments, radiology imaging and imaging reports.
3. Case report forms.
4. Correspondences: Between study sites, IRB, and sponsor on serious adverse events or key issues in the study.
5. Study materials: Protocol, investigator brochure, instructions for use, SAP, and so on.

DATA ANALYSIS

Intention-to-Treat Analysis (ITT)

Analysis by intention-to-treat (ITT) is a strategy that compares study groups in terms of the treatment to which they were randomly allocated, regardless of the treatment they actually received or other trial outcomes. Regardless of protocol deviations and participant compliance or withdrawal, analysis is performed according to the assigned treatment group.[20–22] Thus the ITT strategy generally gives a conservative estimate of the treatment effect compared with what would be expected if there was full compliance. By accepting that noncompliance and protocol deviations are likely to occur in actual clinical practice,[23] ITT essentially tests a treatment policy or strategy, and avoids overoptimistic estimates of the efficacy of an intervention resulting from the removal of noncompliers.

Per-Protocol Analysis (PP)

There is a view that only patients who sufficiently complied with the trial's protocol should be considered in the analysis. Compliance covers exposure to treatment, availability of measurements, and absence of major protocol violations. Such analysis is often referred to as a "per-protocol" or "on treatment" analysis. The main issue arising from this approach is that it might introduce bias related to excluding participants from analysis. Therefore the ITT analysis should always be considered as the ideal primary analysis, possibly supplemented by a secondary analysis using the PP approach. However, if investigators decide differently, their choice must be justified and subjected to strict rules. Examples of protocol deviations that may occur during the course of the study and violate per-protocol analysis are as follows:

- Patients who do not satisfy the inclusion and/or exclusion criteria are included in the trial.
- A patient is randomized to the treatment A but treated with the treatment B.
- Some patients who drop out from the study.
- Some patients who are not compliant, in that they do not take their medications as instructed.

Advantages and Limitations of an Intention-to-Treat (ITT) Analysis

ITT analysis is highly desirable unless there is overwhelming justification for a different analysis policy (e.g., an unacceptably high proportion of ineligible participants).

Advantages

- Retains balance in prognostic factors arising from the original random treatment allocation.
- Gives an unbiased estimate of treatment effect.
- Admits noncompliance and protocol deviations, which reflects a real clinical situation.

Limitations

- Estimate of treatment effect is generally conservative because of dilution due to noncompliance.
- In equivalence trials (attempting to prove that two treatments do not differ by more than a certain amount) this analysis will favor equality of treatments.
- Interpretation becomes difficult if a large proportion of participants cross over to opposite treatment arms.

Requirements for an Ideal ITT Analysis Ideal ITT analysis can be obtained if the following are provided:

- Full compliance with randomized treatment.
- No missing responses.
- Follow-up on all participants.

Subgroup Analysis

Practitioners and regulatory agencies are keen to know whether there are subgroups of trial participants who are more (or less) likely to be helped (or harmed) by the intervention under investigation. Furthermore regulatory guidance strongly encourages appropriate subgroup analyses. The results of subgroup analyses can also drive changes in practice guidelines. For example, the US National Institutes of Health issued a clinical alert following the unexpected finding in the BARI (Bypass Angioplasty Revascularization Investigation) trial that mortality after angioplasty in patients with diabetes was nearly double that after bypass-graft surgery ($p = 0.003$).[24] Meaningful information from subgroup analyses within a randomized trial is restricted by multiplicity of testing and low statistical power. There is therefore a tension between our wish to identify heterogeneity in the responses of trial participants to trial interventions and our technical capacity for doing so. Surveys on the adequacy of the reporting of clinical trials consistently find the reporting of subgroup analysis to be characterized by poor practice.[25–28]

Problems with Subgroup Analysis

The Problem of Multiple Testing Statistical investigation of large numbers of subgroups inevitably shows significant interactions with the effectiveness of the trial intervention. By definition, testing at the 5% level of significance will erroneously report a statistically significant difference between subgroup categories in about 5% of the tests performed (so-called false-positive results). Trials with multiple comparisons to assess the comparability of randomized groups at baseline confirm this prediction.[29,30] In subgroup analyses, where some factors (e.g., sex, age, race, center, smoking status, stage of disease, and coexistent disorders) may influence outcome, the risk of false-positive results is high.[31] Overly enthusiastic analysis of subgroups can reveal statistically significant differences in outcome among subgroups even where neither arm of the study receives any intervention.[32] In some such cases, such as the ISIS-2 study that found a slight adverse impact of aspirin therapy on patients born under the astrological signs Gemini and Libra, and that aspirin helped after the first, but not subsequent, infarctions,[33] the results of the subgroup analysis may be dismissed as contrary to current understanding of biological mechanisms. In other cases, such as the BARI trial,[24] whether the finding of the subgroup is valid can only be established by additional studies.[34,35]

The Problem of Statistical Power   Most studies enroll just enough participants to ensure that the primary hypothesis can be adequately tested. Therefore statistical tests on subgroups have only the power to detect substantially larger effects on the same endpoint. Loss of compliance, together with adjustments for multiple testing, can exacerbate this lack of power.[27] In consequence, when tested separately, many of the subgroups fail to show the statistically significant treatment effect that was shown in the main population; at the same time genuine differences in response to treatment (so-called heterogeneity) among study subpopulations may also go undetected.

Can the Problems be Overcome?   Despite subgroup analyses generally lacking statistical power, when used repeatedly to look for differences across many factors (e.g., sex, age, smoking status, and blood pressure), they tend to detect spurious effects. So some genuine differences may be observed among subgroups on the need to minimize the risk of accepting and publishing false positives.[25,27] One consideration is to accept that the results of subgroup analysis are hypotheses. However, even among experts, opinions range from only accepting prespecified subgroup analyses supported by a very strong a priori biological rationale[36] to a more liberal view by which subgroup analyses, if properly carried out and carefully interpreted, are permitted to play a role in assisting doctors and their patients to choose between treatment options.[37]

Trial Design: Are the Subgroups Appropriately Defined?
Subgroups based on characteristics measured after randomization, such as compliance, should be avoided, since allocation to the subgroup may be influenced by the intervention. Similarly it is preferable to use the intention-to-treat population, since reasons for withdrawal may not be balanced between treatment arms. For example, adverse drug events may be the main factor behind withdrawals from an active treatment arm, the same as lack of efficacy in a placebo-controlled arm.[38]

Important Points to Consider for Subgroup Analyses

- Are the subgroups based on pre-randomization characteristics?
- What is the impact of patient misallocation on the subgroup analysis?
- Is the intention-to-treat population being used in the subgroup analysis?
- Were the subgroups planned a priori?
- Were they planned in response to existing trial or biological data?
- Was the expected direction of the subgroup effect stated a priori?
- Was the trial designed to have adequate power for the proposed subgroup analysis?
- Is the total number of subgroup analyses undertaken declared?
- Are analyses decided on a priori clearly distinguished from those decided on a posteriori?
- Are the statistical tests appropriate for the underlying hypotheses?
- Are tests for heterogeneity (i.e., interaction) statistically significant?
- Are there appropriate adjustments for multiple testing?
- Is appropriate emphasis being placed on the primary outcome of the study?
- Is the validity of the findings of the subgroup analysis discussed in the light of current biological knowledge and the findings from similar trials?

Were the Subgroup Analyses Planned before Commencement of the Study? In general, subgroup analyses should be defined a priori and purposely on the basis of known biological mechanisms or in response to findings in previous studies. Ideally the choice of the subgroups and the expected direction of the subgroup difference should be justified in the trial protocol. Where a particular subgroup analysis is of great interest, adequate power to show the results can be designed into the trial, for example, by using an expanded endpoint for the subgroup analysis. At the other extreme, subgroup analyses that are decided on once the dataset has been examined should be treated with skepticism. Intermediate between these two extremes are cases, such as occurred in the BARI trial in which the subgroup analysis, although not originally planned, was decided on during the course of the trial in response to findings in other studies (with the investigators remaining blinded to the interim results of BARI).[15]

Reporting   The study report should include all the information required to assess the validity of subgroup analyses reported. In particular, the number of subgroup analyses should be declared, as this will enable readers to assess whether the issue of multiple testing is being dealt with. Analyses planned a priori, and the rationale for choosing them, should be clearly stated. Summary data, including event numbers and denominators for all the subgroup analyses, even the uninteresting ones, should be included, as this will facilitate future meta-analyses of the data and help prevent publication bias.[39]

Statistical Analysis   Some investigators avoid the issue of multiplicity of testing by tabulating the observed outcomes for the subgroups of interest without undertaking any formal statistical analysis. The data become available for meta-analysis,[40] but there is the disadvantage that the investigator may fail to detect and draw attention to an important heterogeneity in the population.

The statistical methods used should be appropriate for the hypothesis being tested. The common practice of performing subgroup-specific tests of treatment effect is flawed in that the wrong hypothesis is tested. The hypothesis that should be tested is whether the treatment effect in a subgroup is significantly different from that in the overall population. Testing for a statistically significant treatment effect in a subgroup is hindered by a small sample size.

The appropriate tests to use when analyzing heterogeneity of responses among subgroups are interaction tests. Finally, the article should state whether the statistical tests used included adjustments for multiplicity.

Interpretation of Subgroup Analysis   Because subgroup analyses have less power to detect a therapeutic effect than the main study, the trial report, especially in the abstract or conclusions, should emphasize the overall result. Given the risks of false-positive findings when multiple subgroup analyses are performed, it is not surprising if a subgroup-specific test shows a significant ($p < 0.05$) or suggestive ($p = 0.05$ to $p = 0.10$) effect of treatment, even when the trial failed to do so overall.[25,28] Investigators are often tempted to highlight a particular subgroup analysis.[25,28] For example, in one trial the suggestion that a psychosocial nursing intervention following myocardial infarction was harmful for women ($p = 0.064$), but not for men ($p = 0.94$), was noted, even though the intervention did not affect survival in the overall population[41] (and a test for interaction was not significant[25]). A number of arguments may be used to support the validity of a claimed subgroup effect (e.g., see the BARI trial[24] and Rathore et al.[42]):

- Replication in another independent study.
- Presence of a dose–response relationship.
- Reproducibility of the observation in independent samples within the study, within individual sites.
- Availability of a biological explanation.

Of these parameters, the first could present the strongest evidence. For example, even though the BARI study found no difference in survival following bypass surgery or angioplasty in the overall population, the validity of the subgroup findings was supported by other studies.[24] In another study, the report by Rathore et al. that digoxin use is associated with a significantly increased risk of death among women ($p < 0.014$)[43] was weakened by the fact that it was a post hoc analysis that was motivated by "biological suspicion" rather than by suggestive findings in earlier trials. Biological justifications for the findings of a posteriori (exploratory) analyses, however, carry little weight.[26]

Challenging Issues Due to Subgroup Analysis

It should be noted that when the overall result fails to show efficacy, usually subgroup findings are not acceptable and subgroup analyses at best can be exploratory or hypothesis-generating analyses. When one starts to do multiple subgroups testing, one can easily make a false-positive claim based on such subgroup analysis. We do not know how to interpret the P-values based on such post hoc analysis. Furthermore, without replication of the results in a second well-controlled study, the subgroup analysis cannot be ruled out for a false-positive result.

Although the sponsor may wish to claim approval based on a subgroup of patients, this subgroup hypothesis had to have been stated as a hypothesis of interest to be tested in the original protocol. Any subgroup hypothesis needs to be stated in the protocol, and accordingly proper allocation of α has to be specified. Otherwise, such post hoc subgroup claim will inflate type I error and it is difficult to interpret such p-values.

DATA INTEGRITY

Data quality is attributable to the person who generated the data. Data quality suggests that the data are:

1. Accurate
2. Legible
3. Complete
4. Original

Data integrity refers to the quality of the data overall. Handling of data affects how the study data are maintained, analyzed, and interpreted, and should be detailed in the SAP of the study. In the United States clinical trial data are stored for two years after the market approval of the study; other countries may have different requirements for the data storage time length.

The data management system should be responsible for:

- Case report form (CRF) design, development, and review.
- Standard or customized database design and development.
- Independent data entry, query management, and data quality audits.
- Automatic edit checks to ensure data integrity.
- Routine administrative reporting throughout the study.
- Delivery of clean data files and comprehensive documentation.

CRITERIA FOR USING META-ANALYSIS STUDIES

Clinical research meta-analysis studies are used to support or reject a particular study hypothesis. Ideally the selection of studies requires data to be grouped with similar settings, such as indication, patient population, patient follow-up visits, and endpoints. Since randomized controlled trials are considered the golden mean for clinical trial settings, criteria for using meta-analysis studies could include the exclusion of nonrandomized controlled trials. Clinical outcome endpoints are the preferred endpoints in clinical trials, so nonclinical outcome studies are normally excluded from meta-analysis studies. In addition similar settings among different studies in the meta-analysis process are important. Similar settings include similar follow-up visits, similar outcome endpoints, comparable endpoint time periods, and so forth. The criteria for selecting meta-analysis studies are shown in Figure 2.1.

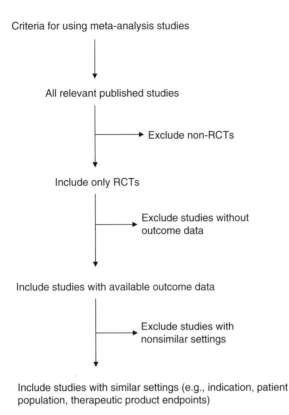

Figure 2.1   Selection of meta-analysis studies

WHO SHOULD HAVE ACCESS TO CLINICAL TRIAL RECORDS

- Sponsor
- IRB/EC
- Regulatory agencies

The following resources are available for maintaining data integrity in clinical studies:

- Guidance for clinical trial sponsors on the establishment and operation of clinical trial data-monitoring committees.
- Updated draft FDA guidance on roles, responsibilities, and operating procedures for data-monitoring committees in overseeing clinical trials.

- Updated FDA guidance giving recommendations for sponsors on submitting information about clinical trials for serious or life-threatening diseases to a data bank.
- Updated Office for Human Research Protections (OHRP) compliance activities.
- OHRP compliance oversight activities on significant findings and concerns of noncompliance.

MANAGING STUDY DATA AND QUALITY ASSURANCE

Managing clinical study data appropriately helps ensure completeness, reliability, and processing of data and so can preserve the integrity of the data. The sponsor is responsible for managing the data generated from clinical trials. Data management should include the following processes, as applicable:

- Data management training for investigators and research staff. The sponsor or his/her representative will provide training to the investigator, and research staff on data management issues, entering data onto CRFs, and so forth.
- Electronic database training if applicable. The sponsor will also responsible for conducting data management training on electronic CRFs if used in the trial.
- Data entry. Entry of data into the database system is validated and managed by the sponsor.
- Database processing of core laboratories and imaging testing centers. The sponsor of the study will manage how data collected from core laboratory and imaging centers are be handled and processed in the study.
- Data management of adverse event reporting. Data management of AE reporting includes coding of AEs, and reporting all aspects of AEs.
- Confidentiality and privacy of data. The confidentiality and privacy of the study data must be managed throughout the trial, for example, by identifying subjects using special ID numbers.
- Database lock. Upon a particular study's completion, the database should be locked (no new data can be entered into the database)
- Database validation. This refers to the methods used to validate the database such as double data entry and validation of the software used.

- Quality assurance measures. Independent audits are used to verify the presence of a quality assurance system (e.g., study monitoring).

The guidelines for monitoring clinical trials for GCP compliance are:

- Identify and define the principles and requirements for GCPs.
- Define the basic roles and responsibilities of the sponsor, the monitor, the investigators, and the FDA as they relate to the quality of clinical trials.
- Understand how GCPs can impact clinical research progress and ensure that GCPs are implemented.
- Clearly put into practice the regulatory, source documentation and record-keeping requirements for clinical trials.
- Ensure that your data and supporting documentation are accurate and presentable for inspection.
- Comply with informed consent and human subject protection requirements.
- Learn how to detect and prevent fraud and misconduct in clinical trials.
- Learn how to manage a FDA GCP inspection.

MISSING DATA ANALYSIS

Examples of Missing Data Analysis—Data Imputation

There are different reasons for missing data in clinical studies. Patients might withdraw from the study, some dropouts due to treatment failures or successes, and others moving their residences. Missing data can have negative effects on the study, ranging from minimal to compromising the outcome of the study when the missing measurements are baseline and follow-up visits. Remember, missing data violate the strict intention-to-treat principal and can impact the per-protocol analysis.

Effects of Missing Data on Study Outcome

Study Power   The success of a clinical study is dependent on measurements that determine the primary outcome of the study. Therefore a reduction in the number in valid assessments available for the primary outcome due to incomplete data can reduce the expected statistical credibility of the study.

Patient Population Subjects who do not complete a clinical study might do so for reasons ranging from treatment failure to extremely good response necessitating no further treatment. These events can greatly diminish the patient population of a study.

Bias The introduction of bias into the study may be due to missing data, such as may affect an estimation of the efficacy of the treatment and the comparability of study groups.

Handling of Missing Data

Imputation of Missing Data When incomplete data cannot be ignored by performing statistical analysis with completed data, the missing, unrecorded data could be imputed. Clearly, this practice can affect the power of the study and introduce bias. Methods of imputation may include the best- and worst-case scenarios of data analysis. The best-case scenario is to impute the missing data from the study; the worst-case scenario is to consider missing data as negative data. Another simple way to impute missing data is to replace the unobserved measurements by values derived from other sources (e.g., other follow-up assessments).

Avoidance of Missing Data[44]

- The best way to deal with missing data is to anticipate patient withdrawals and thus in the design of the study expand the sample size to accommodate for dropouts, subjects lost to follow-up, or withdrawals of consent.
- Sensitivity analysis of missing data is helpful in showing the effects of different missing data on the study results.
- Consider from the start probable best- and worst-case scenarios data analyses.
- Consider previous results of a full set of analyses.

EXAMINATION OF DATA ACROSS STUDY SITES[45]

In device trials, center-to-center variations in a device's effect may be due to a physician's experience or training in using or implanting the device. Other explanation may include variations in patient population, patient management, and reporting practices. A scientifically credible explanation is required to account for any variation of data across study centers. This part of the analysis also becomes important when multi-center trials are conducted and include international sites, so any difference in data across the sites or their quality of the health systems should be accounted for. Furthermore examination of data across study sites will probably have some answers to data that not in line with data from other sites. The variation of data could be due to an extreme situation of extra patients enrolled with more prognostic baseline characteristics than at other sites in the study. The first step in the examination of data across sites is a visual examination of these data; then other complex statistical procedures can used for examine and justify data pooling across study sites. At a minimum, a good scientific explanation is required for data variation from center to center.

Multivariate Analysis[46]

Multivariate, or regression, analysis is used in measuring the impact of variables at points of time for the data set, such as the impacts of age, sex, and baseline prognostic parameters (diabetes, hypertension, etc.) on particular outcomes. Such analysis can help determine certain risk factors in a study. Normalization of these risk factors in study groups eliminates the bias associated with these risk factors.

Examples of Early Termination in Clinical Studies

Early termination of clinical studies usually occurs when results show either an unanticipated major adverse effect or tremendous benefit of the study to the patients. An example of termination due to occurrence of an unanticipated major adverse events is given using the CARET study (a beta carotene and alpha tocopherol study)[47]. The CARET study found an overall increased risk of death from cardiovascular disease for participants taking the supplement. This risk was found to disappear in men soon after beta-carotene use was stopped, although female smokers appeared to have a persistent elevated risk. The intervention phase of the study was stopped two years early when it was found that participants who took the supplements had a 28 percent greater incidence of lung cancer and 17 percent more deaths than the placebo group. The risk of dying of cardiovascular disease was 26 percent higher in supplement users compared to that of the placebo group.

In contrast, the Collaborative Atorvastatin Diabetes Study (CARDS)[49], comparing treatment with atorvastatin (Lipitor®, Pfizer Inc.) with placebo in 2800 patients with type 2 diabetes but without overt heart disease, was halted two years before the planned termination because of a significantly low incidence of fatal and nonfatal coronary events, stroke, and coronary revascularization procedures in the treated patients. The study's interim analysis showed a "substantial and highly significant benefit of treatment."

CHALLENGES TO ADVERSE EVENT REPORTING

Identification on Becoming Aware of an Adverse Event

Instruct Sites in the Protocol on What to Look For The most challenging task when an adverse events occurs is identification by the PI on becoming aware of the event. Most adverse events are identified or discovered during monitoring visits, so the monitor must be experienced enough to identify a suspected adverse event. To facilitate such discovery, the sponsor should instruct the investigators on what to look for in the reporting of AEs, in the protocol or in the investigator's planning brochure. For example, should investigators look for all possible adverse events? Or just report specific adverse events that relate to the study's product or the treated disorder? Are investigators going to report adverse events that related to the disorder? Or do the events need not to be reported? The protocol should specify examples of all possible anticipated AEs. The investigator's brochure is the document that provides more complete background information about the investigational drugs (review of physical, biochemical, pharmaceutical properties, and human metabolism of the product), including the guidance on possible risks of the product.

Information about Collected Adverse Events What type of information need to be reported about AEs?

- Description of adverse event. The description of the adverse event is based on the signs and symptoms of the event. The signs of the event are what the physician sees including the lab and imaging testing and symptoms are what the subject is experiencing. Adverse event are best described when they are based on the signs of the event.
- Extent of seriousness of an adverse event. The determination of whether the AE is serious is based on the identification of one of the components of SAE. Serious adverse events are those events that results in death, a life-threatening condition, hospitalization or

prolonged hospitalization, required intervention to prevent permanent impairment/damage, disability or permanent damage, congenital anomaly/birth defect, and other critical care medical events. A narrative is usually written about every SAE in the study that includes the subject's gender, preexisting risk factors, types of procedure or conditions, the procedure date, descriptions of SAEs, the reasons for the SAEs, event outcomes and resolutions.

· Anticipated adverse event. Anticipated adverse events are those events that are listed in the protocol, IFU, or the Investigator Brochure. Unanticipated device adverse effects (UDAE) are those serious events that are device related but whose frequency or severity is higher to what is mentioned in the protocol.

· Related to study product or study procedure. The relatedness of an adverse event to the study product or procedure should be described whenever is possible by investigators. The cause–effect relationship between the research procedure and the investigational device should be determined by investigators whenever is possible, and also whether a correlation of the product/procedure is unlikely or probable.

· Resolution of adverse event. Time of onset and outcome of adverse event should be recorded. This includes the start date, stop date, or ongoing condition if the adverse event is not resolved. In addition to the outcome of the adverse event, sequelae should be recorded.

· Severity of adverse event. Adverse event should be classified as mild, moderate, or severe:

  Mild. Transient or mild discomfort, no limitation of activity, no medical intervention or therapy is required

  Moderate. Mild to moderate limitation of activity, some assistance may be needed, no or minimal medical intervention or therapy is required

  Severe. Marked limitation in activity, some assistance usually needed, medical intervention/therapy, hospitalization is possible

Serious versus Severe Adverse Events

A severe adverse event may not be considered a serious adverse event. For example a severe headache may not be serious.

Source Documents for AEs   The following source documents are usually used to identify AEs:

- Hospital, physician, and nurses notes
- Patient diaries
- Assessment forms
- Indications for concomitant medication
- Abnormal lab results
- Missed visits
- Reasons for withdrawal or dropout

Review of SAEs

The sponsor of clinical studies is responsible for a review of serious adverse events occurring in the study to determine whether any are SAEs. In certain studies, a blind review process is set up where two independent reviewers review an adverse event in accordance with the protocol and procedures of the study. If there is a discrepancy in the two reviews AE, the event is reviewed by a third independent reviewer, and the opinion of this reviewer overrides the opinions of the other two reviewers regarding the determination of severity.

Adverse Events Analysis

Adverse events occurring during a study are summarized in frequency tables, which give the number of AEs, the number of distinct participants with each type of AE, and AE rates by body system and treatment group. Within each body system category the relative risk of an event (and a 95% confidence interval) is computed for the analyses for the ITT and evaluable analysis datasets.

Instructions Regarding Reporting Time of Adverse Event

Investigators should be instructed about the timing for reporting certain AEs and to whom they should report these AEs.

- The sponsor should specify the timeframe, for example, that investigators must initially report all serious adverse events 24 hours after becoming aware of these events to the sponsor.
- Full written reports should follow to the sponsor within 10 working days of the event.
- Unanticipated adverse device effects (UADE) must be fully reported immediately by the study investigators to the sponsor and

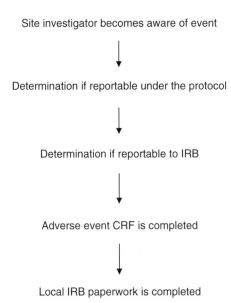

Site investigator becomes aware of event

Determination if reportable under the protocol

Determination if reportable to IRB

Adverse event CRF is completed

Local IRB paperwork is completed

Figure 2.2   Recognition of an adverse event

full written report of these events should be submitted to the sponsor within 10 working days of becoming aware of the event.

- The sponsor must fully report to the FDA, all participating investigators, and all reviewing IRB unanticipated device adverse effects within 10 working days of becoming aware of these events.
- The sponsor should specify whether the SAEs will be reported to the FDA after a specific time period.
- The sponsor should indicate the time period to terminate the study if an adverse event causes unreasonable safety risks to the study patients.
- The sponsor should report serious adverse events to the competent authority in 10 days or as required by each US state or EU member.

Challenges in Reporting Adverse Events

1. Systems that are set up to provide information about an SAE (e.g., MEDWATCH) can lead to underreporting and incomplete reporting during the post-approval phase of the product. MedWatch requires clinicians to recognize that a medical problem may cause an adverse reaction to a product, know how and where to obtain the reporting forms, and invest substantial time writing up the

necessary information. Following through these tasks can lead to substantial underreporting or incomplete reporting.

2. The FDA requires study sponsors or investigators to report an unanticipated problem to the IRB within 10 days. There are many instances of raw and unanalyzed received information that Sails to be reported within the FDA-specified window.

3. With the increase of multinational clinical trials and the huge number of medical products licensed in many countries, companies need to globalize their safety procedures and regulatory reporting.

ADVERSE EVENT CODING SYSTEMS

Several systems for coding of adverse events exist. Two examples are MedDRA (Medical Dictionary for Regulatory Activities) and the ICD-9 (International Classification of Disease Version 9). The MedDRA system is widely used by the FDA for drug studies and is based on the System Organ Class (SOC) heist level of terminology, and distinguished by anatomical or physiological system, etiology, or purpose. Its international medical terminology is designed to support the classification, retrieval, presentation, and communication of medical information throughout the medical product regulatory cycle. For example, the System Organ Class basis of MedDRA for eye disorders takes the form [eye disorders]–higher level group [vision disorders]-higher level [partial loss of vision]–preferred term [vision blurred], lower level term (verbatim) [unable to focus]. Summary tables usually include SOC and preferred terms (percentage of patients with AE). This system can also integrate data from many trials.

The clinical protocol is the document that describes in detail background, purpose, objectives, design, and procedures for the study. A protocol deviation is an unanticipated or unintentional divergence or departure from the expected conduct of an approved study that is not consistent with the current research protocol, consent document or study addenda.

Protocol deviations or violations are divided into serious and non-serious violations.

- Serious violations include the deviations that affect the participant's safety, rights, welfare, or the integrity of the study and the resultant data. Protocol deviations should only be allowed in emergency cases to ensure the safety of the subjects. Specific examples of potentially serious deviations (i.e., that can place subjects at great risk) are improperly obtained informed consents or none obtained, subjects enrolled without meeting eligibility criteria and without prior sponsor approval, study drug or dose not administered per protocol and so increasing the risk of harm to the subject, and unauthorized removal of personal health records off site.

- Nonserious protocol deviations are deviations that do not affect the participant's safety, rights, welfare, or the integrity of the study and the resultant data. Examples of nonserious protocol deviations include missing out-patient visits and study visits made outside the visit window, both cases that do not affect the study outcome.

- Deviation reports are usually forwarded to the IRB at the time of continuing review. The deviation report sent to the IRB should include a description of the protocol deviation and corrective action plan to prevent this from re-occurring. For industry-sponsored studies the sponsor may keep a patient-specific deviation and violation log with each case report form.

- Sometimes protocol deviations are discovered during the monitoring visits of the study. Then the monitoring report should reflect the protocol deviations and corrective action plan to prevent further such violations.

- A protocol violations report must include a description of the protocol violation, notations of any compromise to patient's safety, and documentation of any other safety issues, documentation of the contact with the sponsor on the study's protocol and desired outcome, and a description of the action plan in response to the event.

Examples of protocol deviations include:

1. Changes in procedures initiated to eliminate immediate hazards to study subjects.
2. Enrollment of subjects outside protocol inclusion/exclusion criteria, whether agreed to or not by the sponsor.
3. Medication/intervention errors (i.e., incorrect drug/intervention, incorrect dosage of the drug).
4. Inadvertent deviation in specific research intervention procedures or timing of the research intervention that can affect the safety or efficacy of the study-related intervention or the experimental design.

5. Breach of confidentiality or privacy whereby confidential information about a subject is revealed in inappropriate settings, or to persons without a need to know, or by data exposure (computer security breach, documents left unsecured).
6. Significant deviation from the consenting process.

PROTOCOL DEVIATION REPORT

The protocol deviation report must be completed and signed by the principal investigator or designated representative for the study. The report must include the following items:

1. Description of the deviation with an explanation of the circumstances that led to the deviation and the resulting problem.
2. Whether the deviation did/did not compromise the scientific integrity of the study.
3. Whether the deviation did/did not increase the risk or the possibility of risk for the research subject.
4. Description of the steps taken, or that will be taken, to correct/address the problem resulting from the deviation.
5. Description of a plan to ensure that a similar deviation does not occur in the future.

ADVERSE EVENT REPORTING IN FINAL STUDY CLINICAL REPORT

For the comprehensive analysis of adverse events, all events are analyzed during the research procedure, after short period of procedure completion 7 or 30 days, and during a longer follow-up period of 3, 6, 9, and 12 months or longer. This method of analysis helps determine the relationship between the AE and the product or procedure and also can assist in identifying rare occurring AEs that may be related to the product or procedures in long-term follow-ups.

It should be also determined in the follow-up periods whether the AE is new or continuing, for example, if an AE was described as renal failure after 7 days of procedure (as is supported by an elevation of serum creatinine to <2 mg/dl), and if the same event continues to be observed at 30 days of follow-up. The renal failure is then considered a continuing event and not new AE.

DIFFERENCE BETWEEN THE US AND EU DEFINITIONS AND REPORTING OF ADVERSE EVENTS

US regulations and the EU standard differ in their wording regarding seriousness or severity of an adverse event. The EU regulations (EN 540) address adverse event seriousness based on the adverse event severity grading (mild, moderate, severe, and life threatening). The standard explains that a severe adverse event satisfies almost the same condition listed for a serious adverse event in an FDA IDE study (causes death, hospitalization, prolonged hospitalization, require intervention, results in a congenital anomaly or malignancy, or results in residual damage). The IDE regulations of the United States use the term *serious* as is defined above. Many sponsors try to identify and describe adverse events based on seriousness as well as severity.

ADVERSE EVENT REPORTING CHALLENGES

The following are examples of the challenges in reporting adverse events:

- Adverse events are widely underreported.
- Numerous reports come with inadequate information.
- Investigators have difficulty identifying the specific device involved:
    Patient records remain not documented.
    Devices lack unique identifiers.
    Products undergo frequent modifications.
- Devices that are used as "off-label"
- Devices that shift to home use where nonprofessionals are handling the products.

MINIMIZATION OF BIAS IN CLINICAL TRIALS

Certain procedures or precautions should be undertaken to prevent, or at least minimize, bias in clinical trials:

- Standardize outcome assessments and the use of objective endpoints. The use of objective measurable study primary endpoint(s) is one of the best ways to avoid data evaluator bias (reduction of mortality, increase survival rate, etc.). These endpoints should reflect the clinical outcome of the study as related to the selected subject population. In certain studies surrogate endpoints that reflect the overall clinical outcome may be selected (e.g., lowering blood glucose in diabetic patients, or decreasing blood pressure in hypertensive patients).

- Select an independent study core laboratory for the entire study. This should minimize bias by coordinating interpretations of the test reports, for example, by using the core laboratory for evaluating imaging tests in a study.

- Randomize subjects participating in the study into control (which is given placebo or standard of care therapy) and experimental arms (which is given the investigational product). Randomization is important for achieving equivalent group sizes and for the distribution of any confounder baseline characteristics between the groups.

- Use a double blind design where both the participating subject and the treating physician are blinded to treatment. Blinding is a very effective way of eliminating bias in a trial.

- Use special study committees during the course of the trial, for example, a data safety and monitoring board (DSMB) committee or a clinical event adjudication (CEC) committee. Such committees help ensure that criteria are kept constant during the course of a study in defining serious and major adverse events.

- Evaluate data across study sites for differences in the training and experience of the investigator and the standard of care at each study site.

Selection of Historic Controls

Selection of "historic control" instead of an active control group in medical devices pivotal clinical trials remains a challenging issue in the design of clinical studies. The randomized clinical trial (RCT) is considered the golden standard, but in some circumstances the use of this design may be unnecessary, inappropriate, or even impossible. For example, in certain trials use of randomized clinical studies may raise serious ethical concern because of the risk posed to patients in the control group. Also use of RCT may be discarded if dramatic intervention is called for, such as in life-threatening conditions where at issue is reduction of mortality. Finally, use of RCT is not advised where device effects are to be observed over long follow-up periods, such as with orthopedic implants that require long-term follow-up for use adjustments. Actually, the use of historic controls is considered by the FDA and the scientific community to be the least preferred type of

The Design and Management of Medical Device Clinical Trials: Strategies and Challenges, by Salah Abdel-aleem
Copyright © 2010 John Wiley & Sons, Inc.

control, so this study design should not be used unless there is good evidence to support it. Still the main reason for not using a historic control design is to avoid introducing bias in subject selection and other biases, as will be discussed below. The scientific and regulatory challenges resulting from the use of the historic control can be summarized as follows:

- Erroneous conclusions may be made about the effectiveness of the experimental treatment due to the inherent variability in the historic control data.
- Other challenges are associated with the selection of historic control:

  Absence of historic control data in a reliable and accessible database.

  The sponsor needing to explain thoroughly the scientific arguments supporting the proposed historic control design. If a sponsor elects to use an objective performance criteria approach, the specific literature and rationale justifying this approach should be explained in detail.

  The sponsor needing to provide scientific evidence to match the subject's characteristics of the investigational treatment arm and the historic control arm.

  Information must be given as to whether the historic control was selected from one or multiple studies.

  It must be clarified whether or not the database of selected historic control include detailed individual patient information?

  Information must be given as to whether the selected historic control is validated by new published studies.

Some further important issues regarding the selection of historic control will also be discussed in this chapter: when it might be appropriate to use such noncontrol comparison in medical device pivotal studies, when objective performance criteria (OPC) can be used and what are the advantages and disadvantages for using OPC for historic controls. Additionally this chapter will provide a discussion of recent FDA PMA cases that accept or reject the use of historic controls in clinical studies. It should be noted that concurrent randomized controlled trials are considered the gold standard because this type of study effectively minimizes bias, balance demographics, and supports basic assumptions of standard statistical methodology. The RCT includes a comparison to an experimental treatment, using a group of patients with the same condition, demographics, and prognostic values. Because as many variables as possible are controlled, any differences can be presumed to be due to the new intervention. From the examples of FDA PMA studies that have used historical controls a clear set of recommendations is derived for using historic control in a clinical study and required assumptions are discussed with regard to this type of control.

TYPES OF CONTROL GROUP IN MEDICAL DEVICE CLINICAL TRIALS

The control arm in a clinical study could take the form of the following groups:

1. Randomized controlled trial where patients are randomized into a test group and a placebo group having the same condition, demographic, and prognostic values of the test group.
2. Randomized controlled study where patients are randomized into the test group and an active control group (other treatment).
3. Nonrandomized concurrent control where group of subjects with the same disease or condition have received an intervention (including no intervention) but are separated by time, and usually place, from the population under the current study.
4. Single arm with a historic control where historic control is composed from data of other investigations.

PURPOSE OF CONTROL GROUP

- To distinguish patient outcomes caused by experimental intervention from those caused by natural progression of disease, observer/patient expectations, and other factors unrelated to treatment.
- To make fair comparisons, which is necessary for the study to be informative.
- To draw inferences from the trial.
- To ensure that trial is ethical acceptable.
- To minimize bias in the study.
- To give credibility of the results.

USE OF PLACEBO CONTROL

The "placebo effect" is well known. The placebo control could be no treatment + placebo or standard care + placebo. Matched placebos are necessary so that patients and investigators do not identify which treatment is being used. Trial designers should do their best to match placebo and treatment to prevent patients dropout if patients discover that they are in a placebo program.

ADVANTAGES OF RANDOMIZED CONTROL CLINICAL TRIALS

1. Randomization "tends" to produce *comparable* groups (see Table 3.1).
2. Randomization allows for *valid* statistical tests.

DISADVANTAGES OF RANDOMIZED CONTROL CLINICAL TRIALS

1. Generalizable results. Subjects may not represent the general patient population but rather a volunteer effect.
2. Recruitment. Twice as many new patients may be recruited.
3. Acceptability of randomization process. Some physicians may refuse to participate, and so may some patients.
4. Administrative complexity.

Ethics of Randomization

- Statistician/clinical trialist must benefit from the randomization.
- Physicians should do what they thinks is best for their patients.

TABLE 3.1   Clinical Trial Randomization

Design	Sources of Imbalance
Randomized	Chance
Concurrent (Nonrandomized)	Chance and selection bias
Historic (Nonrandomized)	Chance, selection bias, and time bias

Comparable Treatments

Fundamental Principles of

- Groups must be alike in all important aspects and only differ in the treatment each group receives.
- Technically, "comparable treatment groups" means "alike on average."
- Randomization is used so that each patient has the same chance of receiving any of the treatments under study.
- Allocation of treatments to participants using a chance mechanism results in neither the patient nor the physician knowing in advance which therapy will be assigned, thus blinding patients and physicians to the treatment.
- Psychological influence is absent, enabling a fair evaluation of outcomes.

COMMONLY USED PIVOTAL DESIGNS

- Parallel. Patient is randomized to either treatment (control and experimental).
- Cluster randomization design. Groups (clinics, communities) are randomized to treatment or control.
- Crossover. Patients are randomized to treatment A (control) and treatment B (experimental), but after initiation of the trial patients are allowed to cross over from the control group to experimental treatment.
- Equivalence/noninferiority. Noninferiority trials show that the new treatment is not worse than the standard by more than a defined margin. An equivalence trial is appropriate when it is desired to demonstrate equivalence between two treatments, regimens or interventions (methods) or noninferiority of a new treatment compared to a standard treatment.
- Sequential. Subjects continue to be randomized until the null hypothesis is either rejected or accepted.

Parallel Design

- Hypothesis (H_0): Treatment A versus treatment B.
- Advantages:

Simple, general use

Valid comparison

- Disadvantage: Few questions/study

Crossover Design

Hypothesis (H_0): Treatment A versus treatment B.

- Scheme: Patients are randomized to treatment A (control) and treatment B (experimental) are allowed to cross over from the control group to experimental treatment after initiation of the trial.
- Advantages:

    Each patient able to exercise own judgment

    Smaller sample size

- Disadvantages:

    Not useful for acute disease stage.

    Disease must be stable.

    Assumes no period carryover.

    If carryover, have a study half sized.

Sequential Design

- Subjects continue to be randomized until H_0 is either rejected or accepted.
- Large statistical literature available for classical sequential designs.
- Developed for industrial setting.
- Modified for clinical trials (e.g., Armitage 1975, Sequential Medical Trials)
- Assumptions:

    Acute response

    Paired subjects

    Continuous testing

    Not widely used

Equivalence/Noninferiority

The objective in using an equivalence trial is to rule out differences of clinical importance in the primary outcome between the two treatments. The null hypothesis (in contrast with that in a superiority trial) is stated as a minimum difference that is acceptable and would render the two treatments interchangeable. The execution of an equivalence trial becomes an ambitious exercise because, by necessity, *it requires a much larger sample size than a superiority trial* and is less feasible to conduct.

Noninferiority

Noninferiority trials show that the new treatment is not worse than the standard by more than a defined margin. An equivalence trial is appropriate when it is desired to demonstrate equivalence between two treatments, regimens, or interventions (methods) or noninferiority of a new one compared to a standard treatment. The conduct of an equivalence trial requires different techniques during design and analysis compared to a superiority trial:

- Trial proceeds with active (positive) controls.
- Question is whether new (easier or cheaper) treatment is as good as the current treatment.
- Sponsor must specify margin of "equivalence" or noninferiority.
- Trial cannot statistically prove equivalency, only show that the difference between the treatments is less than something with specified probability.
- Historical evidence of sensitivity must provide to treatment.
- Small sample size, leading to low power and subsequently lack of significant difference, does not imply equivalence.

DEFINITION OF HISTORIC CONTROL

The term "historic control" implies that group of individuals treated in the past and used in a comparison group when the data are analyzed of study that had no control group. The definition implies the following:

- Outcomes of current therapy and patients will be compared against those of previous trials.
- No randomization occurred with regard to current conditions.
- Control group may be too far removed in time.

OBJECTIVE PERFORMANCE CRITERIA (OPC)[48]

Objective performance criteria (OPC) is defined as the criteria agreed upon between the sponsor and FDA to set specific limits to the selected historic control parameters. These criteria are based on broad sets of data from historical databases (e.g., literature or registries) that are generally recognized as acceptable values. These criteria may be used for surrogate or clinical endpoints in demonstrating the safety or effectiveness of a device.

Criteria for OPC

- An OPC is a surrogate for control group but is not an active control group.
- Historical data are derived by pooling different investigations.
- A recognized or agreed-upon acceptable clinical value is fixed with no uncertainty.
- Objective and meaningful standard exists for evaluating the safety and effectiveness of the investigational device to the OPC.
- A benchmark is set for minimally acceptable values.
- Periodical re-evaluation and updating of the OPC is conducted in accordance with the current publications.
- All problems seen with historic controls are considered.

When to Use OPC

The OPC is recommended for use under the following circumstances:

- With well-established standard of care therapy. A great deal is known about the natural history of the disease or condition, and the patient population of the study is well described and relatively stable.
- To gain extensive experience with the investigational device.
- When no safety or effectiveness concern exists about the investigational device.
- With consensus of FDA, industry, clinical, academic, and patient communities.

However, the OPC is not recommended for use under the following circumstances:

- First-in-class devices (e.g., drug-eluting stents).
- New indication sought from the investigational device.
- Unavailability of historic data to the sponsor.
- Inappropriate historic data.

Advantages of OPCs

For the OPC the selected historic control is mainly viewed as an advantage because it can lead to a smaller sample size, reduce risk to the individual patients, provide standard value for all sponsors, and ultimately save time and money; also the study will be easier to execute. The regulatory rational for the use of OPCs in medical devices is included in the scientific evidence in "studies and objective trials without matched controls" (21 CFR 860.7 (c) 92)) "from which it can fairly and responsibly be concluded by qualified experts that there is reasonable assurance of the safety and effectiveness of a device under its condition of use."

Disadvantages of OPCs

The disadvantages associated with OPCs are problems associated with historic control, such as single-arm trials, selection bias, controls regarding data validity and analysis, and smaller sample size studies ($N = 100$ or 150). Additionally sometimes it is very difficult to validate the data of the historic controls.

What Should the Agreement with FDA Contain?[49,50]

The agreement with the FDA regarding the OPC should contain the following:

- Clear definitions of all appropriate terms (e.g., exact numerical value of the control and margin of error).
- Provisions for periodic updating of OPC. The value of the OPC should be periodically updated based on newly published clinical research.
- Specific guidance on methodology to derive an OPC.
- Unambiguous policy regarding failure to meet OPC.

How to Determine OPC?

OPC can be derived from the following sources:

- Past, similar, approved devices.
- Widely accepted OPC Use by clinicians.
- Widely accepted OPC findings in medical literature.

How to Determine Criteria of the OPC

- Rate of OPCs is usually derived from historical data.
- OPCs are usually utilized for noninferior studies.
- The rate of the endpoint (derived from historical control data) + Δ (margin of error).

EXAMPLES OF CLINICAL STUDIES WITH HISTORIC CONTROLS

Three examples of clinical studies that used historic control as the control group are presented in this section. The first study is the laser angioplasty for critical limb ischemia (LACI). The second study is the ARCHeR Registry that the FDA approved regarding carotid stenting device (see Chapter 7). The third example is given using the total artificial heart and left ventricular assist devices.

LACI CLINICAL STUDY

The LACI (laser angioplasty for critical limb ischemia) clinical trial was an IDE study that was designed as a single-arm registry, prospective, and multicenter (US and international sites) study. The design of the study was as follows:

- Patient Population: Patients with critical limb ischemia (CLI) in the Rutherford category 4–6 and considered poor surgical candidates.
- Treatment: Excimer laser atherectomy (ELA) of suprafemoral artery (SFA), popliteal and/or infrapopliteal arteries, with adjunctive percutaneous transluminal angioplasty (PTA) and optional stenting.
- Primary safety endpoint: Any death occurring in six months.
- Primary effectiveness endpoint: Percentage of patients alive without major amputations at six months.

- Study patients were considered poor surgical candidates because of poor or absent vessel for outflow anastamosis, absence of venous conduit, or significant comorbidity.
- Enrollment: 145 patients, 155 limbs at 14 sites in the United States and outside the United States.

The study device was:

- Excimer laser atherectomy
  XeCl excimer laser, 308 nm, pulsed at 40 pulses/second maximum. Delivered via a fiber-optic catheter.
- First approved by FDA in 1993 for use in coronary arteries.

Selection of the Control Group[51]

The control group was selected based on the following criteria:

- Standard of care
- Indicated for LACI treatment
- No ethical implications of substandard care in the control group

Candidate Control Therapies

- Medication (conservative therapy)
- Primary amputation
- PTA + optional stents
- Bypass surgery

Why Randomization Is Not Considered?

Randomization to an appropriate control group could not be achieved because no one therapy of the options listed above was appropriate.

Justification for Selection of Historic Control

Why Not Randomize versus Medications?   Randomizing against a treatment plan that promises 37% major amputation at six months has ethical implications. In the absence of LACI, patients at high risk of surgical mortality would receive medication and bed rest. TASC recommends only prostanoids, and then only when revascularization has failed or is impossible.

Why Not Randomize versus Amputation?   Randomizing against a treatment plan that promises 100% major amputation with a high death rate, both perioperative and long term, raises ethical issues. It might be considered that patients who are not at a high risk of surgical mortality may instead benefit from primary amputation. Yet patients receiving primary amputation are at risk for perioperative mortality, long hospital stay, and high incidence of secondary amputation.

Why Not Randomize versus Bypass?   Bypass surgery is the gold standard for treatment of CLI. However, because LACI patients were poor surgical candidates, bypass was not a treatment option. The reasons why LACI patients were poor surgical candidates are:

- High risk of surgical mortality, and/or
- Missing distal anastomosis site, and/or
- Missing venous conduit for a bypass

Why Not Randomize versus PTA?   Percutaneous transluminal angioplasty (PTA) is not recommended for all disease patterns in critical limb ischemia (see the TASC recommendations). Evidence that PTA can be successful in CLI candidates with poor surgical outcomes is lacking, and is a matter of ethical care in the control group. According to the TASC recommendations, PTA was suitable for the vast majority of patients enrolled in this trial.

Best-Case Historic Control   The following points should be considered when selecting historic control for such a study:

- Exact match in patient characteristics
- Low enrollment number of patients
- Treatment plan that defines the "standard." A mixed set of modalities that uses best-case therapy for each patient.
- TASC recommendations

Historic Control "ICAI Study"   Historic control for the LACI registry was selected from another randomized drug trial treating CLI in 1560 patients: an Italian multicenter study of prostaglandin E1 in CLI patients, with 771 in the alprostadil group and 789 in the control group (published in *Ann Intern Med* 1999; 130:412–21). The control group received variety of therapies (bypass, endarterectomy, medication, and a few PTAs). The study conformed to TASC definitions and GCP.

ICAI Study: Differences ICAI differed from LACI only slightly. ICAI enrolled CLI patients regardless of their candidacy for surgery: 35% of the ICAI patients received surgery as their primary treatment option. LACI, however, enrolled only poor surgical candidates.

Review of Current Consensus

- TASC document recommends PTA for CLI only in simple lesions:
    Type A: single stenoses <1 cm
- TASC does not recommend PTA in:
    Type B: multiple short stenoses.
    Type C: long stenoses; short occlusions.
    Type D: occlusions >2 cm; diffuse disease (surgery is recommended for type D).

TASC Types in LACI About 60% of the patients enrolled in the LACI study were type D (see Table 3.2). Insufficient data were obtained only in 2 out of 155 cases.

Results of the LACI Phase 2 Registry Table 3.3 shows the baseline characteristics of patients enrolled in the LACI study. The only prehistory factor that was significant in the control versus the LACI arm was smokers, whereas prior MI, stroke, diabetes, hypertension, dyslipidemia, and obesity were higher in the LACI arm.

As shown in Table 3.4 patients with high surgical risk were significantly in higher numbers in the LACI arm than the control group.

Planned Criteria For poor surgical candidates the criteria were:

- Rutherford class 4 or higher.
- Absence of suitable autologus vein (SAV) for conduit.
- Extent of pathology.

TABLE 3.2 LACI Lesions as a Function of TASC Lesion Type

TASC Lesion Type	LACI Legs ($N = 155$)
A: short stenoses	3 (2%)
B: multiple short lesions	13 (8%)
C: complex patterns	44 (28%)
D: long diffuse disease	93 (60%)

TABLE 3.3 Patients' Baseline Characteristics

	LACI	Control	p-Value
Mean age, years	72 ± 10	72 ± 10	NS
Men	53%	72%	*
Risk factors			
Smoking current	14%	25%	*
Prior MI	23%	15%	*
Prior stroke	21%	12%	*
Diabetes mellitus	66%	39%	*
Hypertension	83%	49%	*
Dyslipidemia	56%	16%	*
Obesity	35%	7%	*

*Statistically significant.

TABLE 3.4 Lesion Characteristics

	LACI	Control	p-Value
Rutherford category			
4	27%	30%	NS
5 or 6	72%	70%	NS
Reasons for poor surgical candidacy			
Absence of venous graft	32%		
Poor/no distal vessel	68%		
High surgical risk	46%	11%	*
Only one reason	61%		
Any two reasons	33%		
All three reasons	6%		

At actual enrollment the criteria were:

- Only 46% met ASA criteria.
- Only 32% did not have SAV.
- Lesions candidates were 41% SFA, 27% popliteal/tibio-peroneal
    Mean of 2.7 lesions/limb.
    Mean length: 6 ± 7 cm.
- Lesions amenable to PTA

Equivalence Hypothesis The objective was to determine equivalence to historical nonintervention control. The sponsor sought a conservative comparison because LACI patients will be more comorbid

TABLE 3.5   LACI Study Outcomes

Variable	LACI	ICAI
Patients enrolled	145	789
Censored/withdrawn	—	[116]
Patients for analysis	145	673
Lost to follow-up	11 (7.6%)	7 (1.0%)
Patients not lost to follow-up	134	666
Deaths	15 (11.2%)	96 (14.4%)
Alive w/amputation at 6 months	9 (7.6%)	76 (13.3%)
Limb salvage at 6 months	110 (75.9%)	494 (73.4%)
Persisting CLI	43 (29.7%)	211 (31.4%)
Serious AEs	58 (40.0%)	239 (35.5%)
Re-interventions	24 (17.9%)	34 (5.1%)

TABLE 3.6   Primary Effectiveness Endpoint

LACI	Control
75.9% (110/145)	73.4% (494/673)

Note: 95% CI (−5.3%, 10.2%).

and at greater risk for poor outcome. However, the ASA class did not correlate to the risk/benefit of a regional intervention. Only the patient age predicted mortality and the need for amputation (the same in LACI and ICAI studies). In the end it was difficult to determine if one group was sicker than the other, given the differences in risk factors.

The outcome of this study is shown in Table 3.5. The rate of death at six months (11.2% vs. 14.4%), and number of patients alive with amputation at six months (7.6% vs. 13.3%) were lower in the LACI arm compared to the ICAI group. However, the number of SAEs and re-intervention (SAEs 40% vs. 35.5%; re-interventions 17.9% vs. 5.1%) were higher in the LACI arm compared to the historic control group.

Study Design   Because the sponsor desired to show that the results in the treatment group were at least as good as for the control group— an equivalence design—the FDA agreed to accept the equivalence design. FDA acceptance was thus based on the assumption that the control patients would be less sick than the LACI registry patients.

The effectiveness primary endpoint was met as "percentage of alive patients without amputation at six months." Table 3.6 shows the primary effectiveness endpoint: the percentage of alive patients without major amputations at six months.

Limitations of Primary Endpoint of Analysis The primary endpoint was limited by the following factors:

- Nonrandomized design of the study. The visible differences were:
    LACI and control patients not comparable, for example, due to differences in rest pain, previous minor amputations, and previous major amputations.
    Country/hospital factors variations.
- Historical control (raw data at the patient level not available). Visible differences cannot be accounted for because of:
    Absence of raw data
    Formal sensitivity analysis for hidden biases not carried out.
- Missing information.

FDA Panel Discussion

Although the LACI study met the primary endpoints of equivalence in the six-month limb salvage and death rates, the FDA and panel members were concerned that there was not enough evidence to justify from the data the assumption that the patients in the LACI registry would be more comorbid and at greater risk for poor outcome, compared to the control group. The major weaknesses of the selected control were that the selection was based on one study and access to detailed data on patients was not available, which raised concern about the comparability of the patients in the control group and the active test group.

ACCULINK™ and RX ACCULINK™ Carotid Stent System

Selection of the historic control for the ACCULINK™ and the RX ACCULINK ™ carotid stent system is discussed in Chapter 7.

LEFT VENTRICULAR ASSIST DEVICES

Left ventricular assist devices are a class of devices used for life-threatening conditions such as end-stage heart failure. The majority of these trials have been conducted as nonrandomized studies because of the severity of the condition and the ethical issues that it might raise if patients are randomized to standard treatment. Two cardiac assist devices are discussed in this section, the HeartMate II and the CardioWest total artificial heart. In the latter device, even though the FDA questioned the utility of data obtained from the historic or concurrent controls because of noncomparable baseline covariates in the control versus total artificial heart (TAH), ultimately the study was approved by the FDA. The FDA concluded that the efficacy survival to transplant was similar to other devices reported in the literature. Additionally the safety of the device as represented by the adverse event profile trends seem to be similar to other devices, but a direct comparison cannot be made due to differences in definitions.

HeartMate II Left Ventricular Assist System (LVAS)

The HeartMate II LVAS is a left ventricular assist device (LVAD) system, a device that helps the heart's left ventricle deliver blood to the rest of the body. The HeartMate II LVAS includes a pump implanted inside the patient's body and components that remain outside the patient's body. The pump controller and batteries are worn outside the patient's body. The system also includes a battery charger/power supply and monitor that remain outside the body. The HeartMate II pump is implanted below the heart with its inlet attached to the left ventricle and its outlet connected to the aorta. Blood flows from the heart into the pump. A small electric motor in the pump drives a rotor (similar to a propeller) inside the pump that pushes the blood into the aorta and out to the body. A flexible tube passes through the patient's skin and connects the implanted pump to a small controller worn outside the body. The controller is powered either by batteries or connected via a power supply to standard household electrical power outlet. The HeartMate II left ventricular assist system (LVAS) is intended for use as a bridge to transplantation in cardiac transplant candidates at risk of imminent death from nonreversible left ventricular failure. The HeartMate II LVAS is intended for use both inside and outside the hospital or for transportation of ventricular assist device (VAD) patients via ground ambulance, fixed wing aircraft, or helicopter. The HeartMate II LVAS is used in people with advanced (severe) heart failure who are candidates for heart transplantation but are expected to die before a donor heart becomes available. This is often called a "bridge to transplant."

SUMMARY OF CLINICAL STUDIES[52]

Study Overview

Enrolled in the HeartMate II (HMIL) bridge to transplantation (BTT) Primary Study cohort were 126 patients at 26 investigational sites across the United States. The primary objective of the study was to determine, with this pivotal study sample size, the safety and effectiveness of the HeartMate II LVAS as a therapeutic device in end-stage heart failure patients who are listed for cardiac transplant and at imminent risk of death. Effectiveness of the device was assessed on the basis of the percentage of patients surviving either to cardiac transplantation or 180 days of LVAS support, while being listed UNOS IA/IB (listed criteria for mechanical assist devices and the infusion of inotropes). Safety of the HeartMate II LVAS was assessed by the incidence of adverse events during LVAS support. A number of secondary objectives were also evaluated during the study, including clinical reliability (malfunctions/failures), functional status (six-minute walk and patient activity score), quality of life (Minnesota Living with Heart Failure and Kansas City Cardiomyopathy questionnaires), re-operations, neurocognitive assessment (memory, language, visual/spatial perception, processing speed, and abstract/executive function), and 30-day and 180-day post-transplant survival. After completion of enrollment in the primary study cohort, enrollment continued under a continued access protocol (CAP), which was identical to the primary study cohort protocol. Patients who were originally enrolled into these two study cohorts but who had a body surface area (BSA) less than $1.5\,mm^2$ were separated out into a Small BSA patient cohort for analysis.

Study Design

The study was a multicenter, nonblinded, nonrandomized, prospective study. The primary study outcomes were defined as death, cardiac transplantation, device explantation due to myocardial recovery, or survival to 180 days on LVAS support while remaining listed UNOS IA/IB. After reaching the 180-day assessment point, patients continued to be followed until transplantation, explantation, or death. Enrolled were (279) patients at 33 study sites. As shown in Figure 3.1, patients were enrolled in both the primary study cohort and the continued access protocol cohort (CAP). Of the 279 patients enrolled into the three cohorts of the HeartMate II study (Primary Study, Continued Access, and Small BSA), 194 patients were followed to a study outcome point,

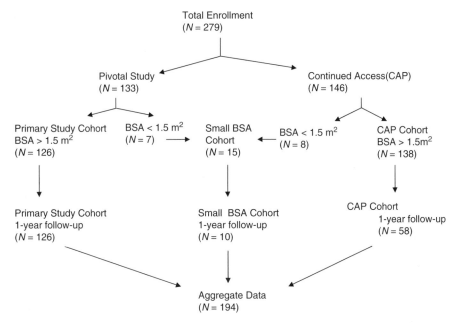

Figure 3.1   Heart Mate II study enrollment chart

and if ongoing on HeartMate II LVAS support, for at least one year. The results are presented in the following clinical summary. As shown in Figure 3.1, the 194 patients are divided among three cohorts; 126 patients in the Primary Study cohort and 58 patients in the Continued Access protocol cohort. An additional 10 patients were originally enrolled in these two cohorts but were separated out for analysis in the Small BSA patient cohort ($1.2 \, m^2 < BSA < 1.5 \, m^2$). Data are presented for each cohort separately and also in the aggregate for all 194 patients.

Patient Population

The patients enrolled into the HeartMate II study were all listed for cardiac transplant in end-stage heart failure and demonstrated no evidence of severe end-organ damage that would make HeartMate II LVAS implantation futile. The inclusion and exclusion criteria were based on study criteria used in previously approved LVAD studies. The criteria included patients with New York Heart Association (NYHA) class IV heart failure, on inotropic support, and without contraindication to be listed for cardiac transplantation as UNOS status IA or IB. Patients who were IB also needed to meet hemodynamic criteria to qualify, including pulmonary capillary wedge pressure (PCWP) or pulmonary artery diastolic pressure (PAD) >20 mmHg and either a cardiac index <2.2 L/min/m^2 or systolic blood pressure <90 mmHg. The study criteria excluded patients with moderately severe end-organ damage, as evidenced by elevated total bilirubin, elevated creatinine values, or low platelet counts, and also excluded patients that may not be able to tolerate the management of the HeartMate II LVAS due to intolerance to anticoagulation or compliance issues.

Table 3.7 shows the baseline characteristics of patient groups by etiology of disease, gender, and patients body surface areas. Table 3.8 lists patients' cardiovascular histories, such as arrhythmia and stroke. Patients' demographics are also provided in Tables 3.7 and 3.8.

Primary Objective

The primary objective of the study was defined as transplant or survival to 180 days for patients listed as UNOS IA/IB.

TABLE 3.7   Patients' Demographics

	Primary Cohort (N = 126)	CAP Cohort (N = 58)	Small BSA Cohort (N = 10)	Aggregate Data (N = 194)
Age (years)[*]	55 (17–68)	56 (16–69)	47 (20–69)	55 (16–69.1)
Etiology	39% Ischemic	50% Ischemic	10% Ischemic	41% Ischemic
Gender	83% Male	78% Male	0% Male	77% Male
	17% Female	22% Female	100% Female	23% Female
MBI (kg/m^2)[*]	26.5 (10–40)	27.6 (18–44)	17.0 (15.6–20.8)	26.6 (15.6–44.0)
BSA (m^2)[*]	1.99 (1.5–2.6)	2.00 (1.52–2.57)	1.40 (1.33–1.47)	1.99 (1.33–2.62)

*Median and range.

TABLE 3.8   Cardiovascular Histories

	Primary Cohort (N = 126)	CAP Cohort (N = 58)	Small BSA Cohort (N = 10)	Aggregate Data (N = 194)
Arrhythmias	101 (80%)	46 (79%)	5 (50%)	152 (78%)
Ventricular Arrhythmias	71 (56%)	34 (59%)	0 (0%)	109 (56%)
Ventricular pacing	77 (61%)	35 (60%)	5 (50%)	117 (60%)
Biventricular pacing	61 (48%)	30 (52%)	0 (0%)	95 (49%)
Implantable cardioverter/ defibrillator	96 (76%)	45 (78%)	6 (60%)	147 (76%)
Stroke	12 (10%)	6 (10%)	1 (10%)	19 (10%)

Overall Patient Outcomes

After reaching the 180-day assessment point, patients continued to be followed until transplantation, explantation, or death. Patient outcomes for each study cohort (Primary, CAP, Small BSA, and Aggregate Data) are presented in Tables 3.9 and 3.10. The prespecified primary endpoint

TABLE 3.9   Primary Study Outcomes

	Primary Cohort (N = 126)	CAP Cohort (N = 58)	Small BSA Cohort (N = 10)	Aggregate Data (N = 194)
Cardiac transplantation	72 (57%)	33 (57%)	7 (70%)	112 (58%)
Myocardial recovery	4 (3%)	2 (3%)	0 (0%)	6 (3%)
Supported >180 days and Listed UNOS status IA or IB[a]	13 (10%)	5 (9%)	0 (0%)	18 (9%)
Not listed status IA or IB[b,c]	9 (7%)	7 (12%)	3 (30%)	19 (10%)
Expired <180 days on LVAD[b]	25 (20%)	11 (19%)	0 (0%)	36 (19%)
Treatment failure; received other VAD[b]	3 (2%)	0 (0%)	0 (0%)	3 (2%)
Prespecified lower 95% confidence Limit of true success rate	65.0%			
Observed lower 95% Confidence limit of study Success rate	64.0%	59.0%	46.2	64.7%

[a]Classified as success per prespecified study criteria.
[b]Classified as failure per prespecified study criteria.
[c]Reasons for not listing included medical ineligibility, elective withdrawal from transplant list, substance abuse, and noncompliance with medical therapy.

TABLE 3.10   Additional Study Results

	Primary Cohort (N = 126)	CAP Cohort (N = 58)	Small BSA Cohort (N = 10)	Aggregate Data (N = 194)
30-Day (perioperative) mortality	12 (10%)	7 (12%)	0 (0%)	19 (10%)
Patient survival to hospital discharge/transplant	105 (83%)	48 (83%)	10 (100%)	163 (84%)
Median time to transplant (days)	102.5	152	194	117
Median duration of device support (days)	117	163.5	374	131.5
Cumulative support duration (patient-years)	71	29	9	109

for the primary study cohort of HeartMate II LVAS pivotal study was "patient survival to cardiac transplantation or 180 days of LVAS support while remaining listed status IA or IB." The HeartMate II pivotal study was to be prospectively determined successful if the one-sided 95% lower confidence limit of the true success rate exceeded 65%, the performance goal. The results show that the lower confidence limit (LCL) of success was 64.0% in the primary study cohort, thereby not quite meeting the prespecified agreed-upon LCL endpoint, >65%.

The primary study outcome is shown in tables 3.9 and 3.10. As shown in these tables the outcomes were similar in the primary cohort and CAP cohort.

FDA Approval Decision

The clinical study results showed that the lower confidence limit (LCL) for the success rate of the prespecified primary endpoint was 64.0% for the HeartMate II LVAS, and the device therefore did not meet the pre-established success criterion of the LCL greater than 65%. The Circulatory System Devices Panel recommended in 2007 that the PMA application be approved because the clinical evidence presented reasonable assurance of safety and effectiveness for the device. FDA reviewed the data supporting the PMA application and determined that even though the true success rate established from the clinical study results was slightly lower than the prespecified primary endpoint, there was sufficient clinical evidence to demonstrate a reasonable assurance of effectiveness for the device in the intended patient population. The clinical study results demonstrated that the HeartMate II LVAS had comparable bridge to transplant success rates as currently approved devices. Similarly patients appeared to have an improved quality of life as well as functional capacity while on the device as confirmed by the improvement in secondary endpoint scores. The incidence of adverse events occurring in patients implanted with the HeartMate II indicated a reasonable assurance of safety. The adverse events experienced were comparable to those seen in previous bridge to transplant trials and reported in the literature. A postapproval study for the HeartMate II LVAS was deemed necessary to assess use of the device outside the clinical trial environment. The postapproval study was also to collect data on the use of the device in smaller size patients, gender-specific outcomes, and peri- and postoperative management of hemorrhagic and thrombotic events.

CardioWest Total Artificial Heart

Study Objective The study aimed to demonstrate that the CardioWest Total Artificial Heart (TAH-t) is safe and effective in providing circulatory support as a bridge to cardiac transplantation in patients with biventricular failure. Bridge to transplant is defined as the use of a circulatory support device to maintain viability for transplantation until a donor organ is procured.

Study Design The study was approved under IDE G9201 01 as a nonrandomized, multicentered trial with both historic and concurrent controls. Patients were transplant candidates who were at risk of imminent death from biventricular heart failure. The overall objective of this study was to determine if the TAH-t was safe and effective for bridging patients to cardiac transplantation. A total of 95 patients were enrolled. Of these, 81 formed the core implant group and an additional 14 patients did not meet study entrance criteria and were considered an out-of-protocol cohort, treated under compassionate use. IRB acknowledgments were obtained for each patient. The data used to demonstrate safety and effectiveness were collected from patients enrolled at five US investigational sites.

Effectiveness Parameters Treatment success was defined as patients who, at 30 days posttransplant, were:

- Alive
- New York Heart Association class I or II
- Not bedridden
- Not ventilator dependent
- Not requiring dialysis

Overall survival, hemodynamics, kidney, and liver end-organ functions were secondary effectiveness endpoints.

Safety Parameters Patients were clinically assessed and adverse events were evaluated for safety.

Study Protocol

Inclusion Criteria Patients who met all of the following inclusion criteria were eligible for the study:

- Signed informed consent
- Eligible for transplant
- New York Heart Association functional level IV

Exclusion Criteria   Patients with any of the following conditions were excluded from the study:

- Use of any ventricular assist device
- Pulmonary vascular resistance >8 Wood (640 Dynes-s/cm)
- Dialysis in previous 7 days
- Serum creatinine >5 mg/dl
- Cirrhosis with bilirubin >5 mg/dl
- Cytotoxic antibody >10%

Treatment Procedures   All patients were screened for study eligibility. The treatment group met eligibility criteria within 48 hours of the implant procedure, signed an informed consent and received a TAH-t implant.

Term of Study   Patients were followed through the primary endpoint of 30 days posttransplant, and then monitored for survival annually.

Hemodynamic Insufficiency Demonstrated by A or B Below

- Cardiac index <2.0/mini/M^2 and one of the following:
    Systolic arterial pressure <90 mmHg
    Central venous pressure >18 mmHg
- Two of the following:
    Dopamine >10 p.g/kg/min
    Dobutamine >10 p.g/kg/min
    Epinephrine >2 p.g/kg/min
    Isoproterinol >2 kg/kg/min
    Amrinone >10 μg/kg/min
    Other drugs at maximum levels
    Intra-aortic balloon pump (IAPB)
    Cardiopulmonary bypass (CPB)

Comparison Population   A comparison group was initially identified by retrospective review during a time period when the TAH-t was not available to the participating centers. Analysis of the baseline data from this group of patients revealed that they were not comparable to the treatment group. An imbalance in the year of implant and in multiple baseline covariates made statistical comparisons inappropriate. Therefore a survival to transplant performance goal (65%) that had been developed for bridge to transplant in univentricular devices (LVADs) was used as a guideline. It should be noted that the adverse events were not compared to a performance goal due to different definitions. The LVAD performance goal was established from a literature search of articles published in 1997 or after for the bridge to transplant indication. The criteria for inclusion were at least 20 adult patients, original data, wide geographic distribution, and enough detailed data to determine the results in LVAD adult patients. The criteria for exclusion were duplicate papers reporting the same population, registries, meta-analyses, RV support at initial implant, and cardiogenic shock patients.

Table 3.11 shows the mean time to cardiac transplant or death. The mean core patient wait for a donor heart was 79 days, with a median wait time of 47 days. The clinical trial outcomes are shown in Table 3.12, including survival to transplant and survival to 30 days posttransplant. At 30 days posttransplant, 69.1% (56/81) of the core implant group met the criteria for treatment success.

The primary endpoint of the study was treatment success. To be considered a success, the patient had to have been, at 30-days posttransplantation, (1) alive, (2) NYHA class I or II, (3) ambulatory,

TABLE 3.11 Time to Transplant or Death

Time	Statistic	Core ($N = 81$)
Duration (days)	Mean (SD)	79.1 (83.9)
	Median	47.0
	Min–max	1.0–414.0

TABLE 3.12 Clinical Trial Outcomes of Core Patients

Outcome (95% CI)	Core Patients ($N = 81$)
Survived to transplant	64 (79%) (68.5%–87.3%)
Survived to 30 days posttransplant	58 (71.6%) (60.5%–81.1%)
Treatment success (30 days posttransplant)	56 (69.1%) (57.9%–78.9%)

(4) not ventilator dependent, and (5) not on dialysis. Patients who failed these criteria were considered failures with respect to the study. At 30 days posttransplant, 69.1% (56/81) of the core implant group met the criteria for treatment success.

The Circulatory System Devices Panel recommended that the SynCardia System's PMA for the SynCardia Systems, Inc. CardioWest temporary Total Artificial Heart (TAH-t) be approved. The FDA concurred with the panel's recommendation.

SUMMARY OF RECOMMENDATIONS FOR HISTORIC CONTROLS

The following recommendations are provided for trial sponsors when they are considering use of historic control in a clinical trial:

1. Historic control is mainly selected if randomization to the control group raises ethical concerns because of risks associated with patients in the control group.
   a. Trials designed to treat life-threatening conditions.
   b. Benefit of the investigational device could be dramatic.
   c. Investigational therapy could have a dramatic effect in reducing mortality.
2. Historic control data from a reliable detailed database can provide information on comparison parameters.
3. If possible, the historic control data should be obtained from multiple studies or multiple databases.
4. It is important to validate the historic control data as new studies are published.
5. Patients' baseline characteristics in the proposed study and in the historic control group should be comparable.
6. If the historic control is based on international studies, then country and hospital factors should be considered.
7. Historic controls can be used in certain circumstances if the following information is available:
   a. Much is known about the natural history of the disease or condition.
   b. Underlying patient population is well described and relatively stable.

    c. Extensive clinical history and experience are provided with the device.

    d. Standard of care are well known.

    e. No significant new questions of safety or effectiveness are raised.

    f. Consensus exists among FDA, industry, clinical, academic, and patient communities about the selected historic control.

8. Study sponsor's should agree with the FDA regarding the OPC for the historic control:

    a. Clear definitions should be given of all technical terms.

    b. Provisions are made for periodic updating of the OPC.

    c. Specific guidance is available on methodology used to derive an OPC.

    d. Unambiguous policy is in place regarding failure to meet the OPC.

CHAPTER 4

Fraud and Misconduct in Clinical Trials

Fraud and misconduct in clinical research is any intentional and serious deviation from acceptable practices such as fabrication, falsification, and plagiarism. When looking for misconduct, it must be distinguished between (1) innocent ignorance and lack of knowledge, (2) sloppiness, and (3) malicious intent. An example of malicious intent is creating patients and/or creating data. A noncompliance based on lack of regulatory knowledge may be highlighted in the following example: backdating the subject signature on an ICF because the subject forgot to put the date on the form originally and the study monitor is coming to monitor the study soon. Misconduct of sloppy kind due to inadequate staff, or lack of supervision may include the following examples: lack of obtaining ICF from subjects, and protocol ignored and shortcuts taken. However, the most serious misconduct issues are represented in the malicious misconduct in the following examples: recording subjects that were never enrolled in the trial, creating data that were never obtained, or substituting the study data with different data.

This chapter discusses fraud and misconduct issues in clinical studies. Although fraud occurs at rare percentage, the sponsor should be aware

The Design and Management of Medical Device Clinical Trials: Strategies and Challenges, by Salah Abdel-aleem
Copyright © 2010 John Wiley & Sons, Inc.

of any fraud or misconduct in clinical trials and must take the necessary precautions to deal with these issues in timely and efficient manner. In this chapter the following issues are addressed: definition of fraud, its consequences, its warning signs, fraud prevention, and to whom fraud should be reported. A set of tips are provided for detecting serious misconduct.

The reader of this book will gain experience in detecting, correcting, and preventing clinical study misconduct and fraud at domestic and international clinical sites. Additionally readers will learn how to ensure that their study conduct and supporting documentation is accurate and factual. The chapter will also address how to uncover misconduct, as well as how to deal with its consequences while identifying proactive solutions to prevent further problems.

The chapter will further cover methods to detect misconduct and deal with fraud in clinical trials by defining the basic requirements of good clinical practices (GCP):

- Appropriate duties and oversight required of the sponsor, monitor, and investigators to ensure a high level of quality in a clinical trial.
- Quality practices designed and implemented to guarantee complaint clinical trials.
- Techniques used to uncover and preclude fraud and misconduct in clinical trials.

It should be noted that falsification places subjects in the trial at possible risk, and jeopardize the reliability of submitted data. Investigators who are involved in misconduct could be subjected to disqualification, debarment, or prosecution by the FDA. Sponsors could be subject to data exclusion, debarment, or prosecution.

FRAUD AND MISCONDUCT IN CLINICAL TRIALS[53–55]

It is difficult to determine fraud in clinical trials, but this phenomenon is still considered rare. Approximately 3% of FDA inspections uncover serious GCP violations resulting in warning letters.

Definitions of Fraud

Research misconduct means fabrication or falsification in proposing, designing, performing, recording, or reviewing research, or in reporting research results. Research misconduct does not include honest error or honest differences of opinion.

Who Commits Fraud?

Any of the following entities could commit fraud: investigators, study coordinators, data management personnel, lab personnel, IRB staff, CRAs and sponsor personnel, and FDA.

Consequences of Fraud

Fraud has several negative impacts on the sponsor, investigator, study institution, and study subjects:

- *Sponsor.* Data validity compromised, regulatory submission jeopardized, additional costs.
- *Investigator.* Fines, legal expenses, disqualification/FDA debarment, license revocation, incarceration, ruined career.
- *Institution.* Lawsuits against study institution.
- *Subject.* Safety at risk, loss of trust in clinical trial process.

Why Does Fraud Occur?

Fraud may happen as a result of lacking resources (staff, time, and subjects), no GCP training, no regulatory oversight, pressure to perform or to publish, or for monetary gain or greed.

WARNING SIGNS OF FRAUD

There are several warning signs of fraud, for example, high staff turnover; disgruntled staff because of a fearful, anxious, depressed, defensive, and high-pressure work environment; absent investigators; lack of GCP training; or pressure for highly unusual fast recruitment.

Data Identifier Signs of Fraud

The following are data identifiers of fraud:

- Trends/patterns not plausible:
    100% drug compliance.
    Identical lab/ECG results.

No SAEs reported in study where SAEs are expected.

Subjects adhering perfectly to a visit schedule.

Perfect efficacy responses for all subjects.

- Site data not consistent with other centers (statistical outlier) despite the absence of any training need for the site.
- Source records do not show an audit trail. No signatures and dates of persons completing documentation are available.
- Perfect diary cards, immaculate CRFs, are presented.
- Subjects[1] handwriting and signatures are inconsistent across documents (consents, diaries).
- Questionable subject visit dates are noted (Sundays, holidays, staff vacations).
- Impossible events are recorded (e.g., subject randomized before IP even available at the site).
- Subject visits cannot be verified in the medical chart or appointment schedule.

TIPS FOR DETECTING SERIOUS MISCONDUCT

- Get Technical-Read and evaluate X rays, EKGs, and lab results. Don't just inventory the source document.
- Ask study monitor to see the patient's medical chart to prevent violations from going undetected.
- Fill in the blanks, that is, question missing dates, times, information, and offer to retrieve records.
- Don't be intimidated.
- Believe the monitor, and put the burden of proof on the clinical investigator.
- Be suspicious of blame shifting. Tell the clinical investigator he/she is responsible for the conduct of the study and is accountable for the results.
- Cultivate whistleblowers. Establish rapport with study staff, be approachable and available, listen to grievances, and observe working conditions.

FALSE CLAIMS ACT

- It is unlawful to submit a false or fraudulent claim for payment to the US government.

- Private citizens who know of people or companies defrauding the government may sue on the government's behalf.
- The plaintiff shares in the proceeds of the suit.
- Protection is assured for whistleblowers who are harassed, threatened, discharged or otherwise discriminated against in their employment.

FRAUD PREVENTION

The following recommendations are provided to prevent fraud:

- During pre-study evaluation, sponsors should carefully scrutinize sites for interest in the study, stability of the staff, investigator/staff interactions, workload, and level of training.
- Everyone involved in the clinical trial process should complete regular GCP training.
- CRAs should be expert on the protocol, particularly with parameters that determine eligibility (inclusion/exclusion criteria), adverse event reporting, and primary efficacy and safety endpoints.
- Sponsors should emphasize their rules for study adherence at the initiation visit.
- Institutions should set up systems to encourage fraud reporting and protect whistleblowers.

POLICY ON HANDLING COMPLAINTS OF MISCONDUCT

- All complaints should be assumed to be credible unless demonstrated to the contrary after thorough evaluation and supervisory review.
- All decisions on the follow-up action required for a complaint should have documented supervisory review and approval.
- All complaints should be documented and evaluated for follow-up upon receipt.
- Complaints requiring action should be followed up as soon as possible.
- Identify complaints that will be followed up on a high priority basis, such as reports of gross abuse of subjects' rights that result or have the potential to result in death or injury, reports of fraud, falsification, or other criminal activity.

- Assign due date to ensure that complaints are evaluated and acted on immediately.
- The receipt, follow-up, and action on all complaints should be documented from cradle to grave so that all decisions and actions can be reconstructed from the complaint-handling documentation.

REPORTING RESEARCH MISCONDUCT

The following information is needed to report misconduct:

- Name of the person(s)
- Contact information
- Specific identity of the affected research
    IND/IDE number, protocol, study title, and study dates
    All information on the research misconduct available to the sponsor
    Timely sharing of information on problem investigators
    Amended Privacy Act notice
    Bioresearch Monitoring Information System (BMIS)/ CI inspection list
    Misconduct websites

BIORESEARCH MONITORING INFORMATION SYSTEM (BMIS)

- The bioresearch monitoring information system (BMIS) lists all clinical investigators, CROs, and IRBs involved in the conduct of investigational new drug studies with human investigational drugs
- Information is abstracted from FDA Forms 1571 and 1572, or other pertinent IND submission documents (CVs, cover letters, investigator lists).
- File contains a separate entry for each time an investigator, CRO, or IRB is identified in a new submission (i.e., if an investigator is named in 10 INDs, his/her name will appear 10 times in this file).

Misconduct Website FDA Homepage

- www.fda.gov/ora/compliance.ref/default.htm
- FDA Debarment list

- Disqualified/Restricted/Assurances list
- PHS Administrative Actions list

Where to Report Misconduct

Drugs   Division of Scientific Investigations (HFD-45), Office of Medical Policy, Center for Drug Evaluation and Research, FDA, 7520 Standish Place, Room 103, Rockville, Maryland 20855-2773, (301) 594-0020, fax (301) 594-1204.

Biological Products   Office of Compliance and Biologics Quality, Division of Inspections and Surveillance, Center for Biologics Evaluation and Research, (HFM-650), FDA, 1401 Rockville Pike, Room 400S, Rockville, Maryland 20852-1448, (301) 827-6221, fax (301) 443-6748.

Medical Devices   Office of Compliance, Division of Bioresearch nni-toring, (HFZ-310), Center for Devices and Radiological Health, FDA, 2098 Gaither, Room 130, Rockville, Maryland 20850, (301) 594-4718, fax (301) 594-4731.

CHAPTER 5

Challenges to the Regulation of Medical Device

When designing a clinical trial for a medical device it is useful to consider both regulatory requirements and the sponsor's marketplace objectives. The FDA is concerned about the ultimate safety and effectiveness of the product. However, the sponsor and financial investors are interested in comparative performance, superiority, and product differentiation claims.

Medical devices are increasingly complex and many are critical to sustaining life. All medical devices must meet stringent standards set by the FDA, so the device manufacturer must provide procedures and tests that prove the safety and effectiveness of the device. Obtaining this information is complicated by the fact that the pathway from product design to product launch for a new medical device is often not direct, for a number of challenges and questions often arise, making the final medical device considerably more complex than at first envisoned. In addition the designer must keep up with new emerging

The Design and Management of Medical Device Clinical Trials: Strategies and Challenges, by Salah Abdel-aleem

standards as well as know the ones already in place, and devices using different standards must be made compatible with central management systems.

Among the regulatory challenges to the medical device classification and submission discussed in this chapter is the process of 510(K) premarket notification. It is up to the sponsor to determine why its device should be identified as a 510(K) device. The notion of a 510(K) "substantial equivalence" is addressed and clarified.

Regulations pertaining to the IDE process are also discussed in this chapter. Since the sponsor is the entity responsible for the initial determination of non-risk devices, recommendations are given to the sponsor on how to complete this task, and the requirements for nonsignificant risk device determination are explained. The similarities and difference of the regulations between medical devices and drugs are listed to allow the reader to see these differences and recognize the complexity of pre-clinical and clinical issues in drug and medical device developments. A comprehensive evaluation of the difference between drugs and medical device is given in this section.

This chapter also provides an introduction to the development of combination products, on how these products are determined as combination products, on sponsor–FDA meetings, and on how the sponsor can best use the opportunity of meeting with the FDA to gain required information. Because combination products are becoming ever more complex, tips are given on how to determine a combination product and how to seek the FDA advice regarding this issue. Issues pertaining to time, preparation, and outcomes of FDA–sponsor meetings are covered at the end of the chapter.

DETERMINATION OF 510(K) DEVICES

510(k) is a Premarket Notification submission and allows the manufacturer to demonstrate that the device is substantially equivalent to a currently marketed predicate device at least in one of these parameters:

- Materials
- Design
- Technology
- Intended use
- Performance device

Substantial Equivalence: could establish that the device has the same intended use as a legally marketed predicate and:

1. The same technological characteristics; or
2. Different technological characteristics, but is as safe and effective as a legally marketed device; and
3. Does not raise different questions of safety or effectiveness

The specific information needs to be in the 510 submission could be summarized as follow:

- **Substantive information requirements**
  - Introduction/background
  - General device information
  - Classification name
  - Common/usual name
  - Trade/proprietary name
  - Product code
  - Classification
  - Regulation number
  - Panel

Device sponsor information

- Sponsor name
- Sponsor address
- Establishment registration number (if any)
- Official correspondent
- Performance standards (if any)
- Device description
- Drawings/photographs

Predicate device information

- Predicate name
- Predicate indications for use
- Substantial equivalence
- Statement of similarities to and differences from predicate

Performance data

- Software
- Bio compatibility
- Packaging
- Sterilization
- Shelf life
- Labeling
- Proposed device
- Predicate device
- Confidentiality
- Class III summary and certification (if needed)
- Appendices, as needed

- **510(k) summary (or 510(k) statement)**

    510(k) Summary:

    Must include sufficient detail to provide basis for substantial equivalence determination

    510(k) Statement:

    Certified statement agreeing to provide a copy of non-confidential portions of 510(k) within 30 days of request from anyone

- **Confidential treatment of information in 510(k)**
    - Nothing released during device review process
    - Trade secret and confidential commercial information is not released
    - Once cleared by order, 510(k) information available through Freedom of Information Act (FOIA) request if a 510(k) summary is submitted, will be available on FDA website shortly after clearance is granted

- **Financial disclosure requirements for clinical investigators**

    Applicants are required to either:

    a) Certify that no significant financial arrangements exist between the clinical investigator and the study sponsor (FDA form 3454); or

    b) Disclose to the FDA the nature of the financial arrangement (FDA form 3455) includes: compensation, proprietary interest and significant payments in kind (such as stocks, grants, honorarium, equipment) in excess of 25 k

The 510(K)-premarket notification substantial equivalence could be based on the terms of safety & effectiveness to a predicate device and/

or with respect to intended use and design approval. The 510(k) pre-market notifications require 90-day review cycle by FDA and may also require the inclusion of data from clinical studies.

510(K) "SUBSTANTIAL EQUIVALENCE DECISION MAKING PROCESS"

The Process of 510 K "substantial equivalence decision making process" need to be followed carefully to compare new devices to marketed devices. FDA requires additional information if the relationship between marketed and "predicate" (pre-amendments or reclassified post-amendments) devices is unclear. The decision to whether the new device is substantially equivalent to a predicate device or not, depends on two main questions: Does the new device have the same indication statement? Does the new device have the same technological characteristics, e.g., design, materials, etc.?

Because all new devices, which haven't predicate devices, are usually placed in Class III, the sponsor may utilize the strategy of De Novo review re-classification if they believe that their device have low risk within 30 days of receive of the letter. To qualify for De Novo re-classification, the device should be novel and low risk. The sponsor should submit information that will support their recommendation (bench, animal, and human data). FDA has 60 days to review the petition. FDA could classify the device as Class I, II, or determines that the device should be Class III.

DETERMINATION OF NON-SIGNIFICANT RISK DEVICES (NSR)

The assessment of whether or not a device presents a non-significant risk device (NSR) is initially made by the sponsor and then confirmed by corresponding IRB that may agree or disagree with the sponsor's initial NSR assessment. The IRB serves, in a sense, as the FDA's surrogate with respect to review and approval of NSR studies. If the reviewing IRB agrees with the sponsor's designation of a device study as NSR, the investigation may begin at that institution immediately, without an IDE application approval by the FDA.

Non-significant risk studies must follow abbreviated IDE regulations (21 CFR 812.2(b))

· IRB approval
· Labeling
· Informed consent

- Monitoring and records
- Prohibition against promotion

To be classified as a Significant Risk (SR) device, it must include one of the following features:

- Present a potential for serious risk to subject health, safety, or welfare
- Intended as an implant

Used in supporting or sustaining human life

Difference between PMA Approval and 510 k Clearance

In order for PMA to be approved, a PMA must demonstrate "reasonable assurance" of a device's safety and effectiveness, an inquiry that entails weighing "any probable benefit to health from the use of the device against any probable risk of injury or illness from such use." [*See* FDC Act § 513(a)(1)(C), (a)(2)(C)]. Whereas, devices subject to 510(k) review, are not held to the PMA standard of proof of safety and effectiveness in the first instance. Rather, such devices are held to standard of "substantial equivalence to a predicate device, i.e., a legally marketed pre-MDA device. The term "substantially equivalent" or "substantial equivalence" means, with respect to a device being compared to a predicate device, that the device has the same intended use as the predicate device.

Predicate "creep" is a phenomenon peculiar to the 510(k) program: minor differences among successive device predicates accumulate so that even if a device and its immediate predicate are similar, the last cleared predicate and the generic type of device described in the classification regulation can be made from different materials, use different sources, and have indications for different anatomical sites. FDA states that the submission must include data to support a required statement indicating the device is similar to and/or different from predicates. CDRH requires clinical data in some 510(k)s for devices with different indications from identified predicates.

SIMILARITIES AND DIFFERENCES BETWEEN MEDICAL DEVICE AND DRUG REGULATIONS IN CLINICAL TRIALS

Drugs and medical devices has several similarities and differences by nature of the clinical development process and the mechanism of action of a product. A common regulatory goal is that the market approval of a product be based on providing evidence for its safety and efficacy.

Pre-clinical, clinical, and regulatory differences between drugs and medical devices can exist in the following areas:

- Type of product
- Product classification
- Mechanism of action
- Product development
- Length of time and available funds
- Preclinical differences
- Different regulatory pathways for product approval
- Clinical trial design differences
- Postapproval differences

Type of Product

DEFINITIONS OF DRUGS AND DEVICES

Drugs   Drugs may be defined as substances that:

- Are intended to diagnose, cure, mitigate, treat, or prevent disease.
- Affect the structure and function of the human body.
- Are ingested not as food but as listed in the US Pharmacopoeia, US Homoeopathic Pharmacopoeia, or National Formulary.

Devices   Whereas devices can be defined as mechanisms that:

- Do not achieve primary effect through chemical action.
- Are not dependent on being metabolized.
- Can include device/drug and device/biologic combinations.
- Are classified based on the level of risk and required controls involved.
- Can be an instrument, apparatus, implement, machine, implant, or in vitro reagent as listed in the US Pharmacopoeia or National Formulary.

It should be noted that combination devices such as drug-eluting stents are excluded from these definitions because these products have some characteristics of both devices and drugs.

Device Classification

Medical devices are classified into three classes in accordance with the risks associated with using the devices, whether the device is used to treat a life-threatening condition, and whether the device need to be implanted inside the body.

Class I (General Controls)   Examples are elastic bandages, examination gloves, and hand-held surgical instruments

- Are low-risk devices that call for general controls only, with emphasis on reasonable assurance of the safety and effectiveness.
- Require 510(K) application if they are not exempt.
- Are often simpler in design than class II or III.

Class II (General Controls and Special Controls)   Examples are powered wheelchairs, infusion pumps, and surgical drapes.

- Require more regulatory control than class I.
- Require special labeling, mandatory performance standards, and postmarket surveillance.

Class III (Premarket Approval)   Examples are replacement heart valves, silicone gel-filled breast implants, and implanted cerebella stimulators.

- Require stringent regulatory oversight and sufficient evidence to assure safety and effectiveness.
- Be intended to support or sustain human life, and substantially to be involved in preventing impairment of human health, or presenting a potential or unreasonable risk of illness or injury.
- Require clinical data and premarket approval.

From this classification it is clear that medical devices require more training for investigators than drugs, particularly the class III devices.

Mechanism of Action

Devices and drugs have different mechanisms of action:

- Local device versus drug systemic effects.
- Physical effects for devices versus pharmacokinetic effects of drugs.

Length of Time and Available Funds

In general the process of drug development requires more time and funds than that of medical devices. The drug development process requires Pre-clinical, clinical development (Phase I, II, and III), FDA approval, and post-market approval phase. This process may take an average of 20 years. On the other hand, the device development process requires design of the product, pre-clinical testing, human clinical trials (feasibility and pivotal studies), FDA approval, and may also require post-market evaluation. This Process takes an average of 6-10 years.

Different Regulatory Pathways for Product Approval

Drugs and devices are both regulated by the US Food and Drug Administration. The FDA regulation of drugs started earlier than devices (1938 for drugs, 1976 for devices). Drugs are regulated by the Center for Drug Evaluation and Research (CDER) and regulated by 21 CFR part *312* (investigational drugs) and 21 CFR part *314* (market approval). Devices are regulated by the Center for Devices and Radiological Health (CDRH) and regulated by 21 CFR part *812* (investigational devices) and 21 CFR part *814* (market approval). However, the following regulations are common to both drugs and devices: 21 CFR part 50 (protection of human subjects), 21 CFR part 56 (institutional review boards), 21 CFR part 54 (financial disclosure), 21 CFR part 11 (electronic records), and HIPAA privacy rule.

Investigational Product Applications

Drugs (part 312)

- Investigational New Drug (IND) submitted prior to conducting a clinical investigation with an investigational drug (312.20).
- Exemptions (312.2b).

Devices (part 812)

- Investigational Device Exemption (IDE) submitted prior to conducting a clinical investigation (812.20).
- Two different paths for significant and nonsignificant risk devices:
  Significant risk devices require the approval of the FDA prior to conducting the study.

Nonsignificant risk devices do not require the approval of the FDA prior to conducting the study

- Exemptions (812.2c):

    To obtain exemption from federal law on prohibiting shipment of an unapproved drug or device in interstate commerce.

    To obtain a permit use product in a clinical study to collect safety and efficacy data.

IND exemptions and IDE exemptions may include the following parameters:

IND Exemptions

- Lawfully marketed in the United States
- Not intended to support a new indication.
- Not intended to support a change in advertising.
- Not to involve a factor that increases risk of use.
- Conducted in compliance with IRB (part 56) and Informed Consent (part 50) requirements.
- Compliance with the requirements for promotion and charging of investigational drugs (312.7)

IDE Exemptions

- Use in accordance with indications.
- Noninvasive diagnostic.
- Consumer preference testing.
- Solely for veterinary use.
- Research on or with lab animals.
- Custom device (not being used to determine safety and efficacy for commercial distribution).

IDE Decision Process   Figure 5.1 shows the classification of medical devices as significant and nonsignificant devices compared with IDE exempted devices. The IDE devices require prior approval of the FDA before the start of an IDE study. The abbreviated IDE (A-IDE) devices do not require FDA approval before an A-IDE study is initiated but do require IRB approval.

IND Content   The IND application contains the following contents:

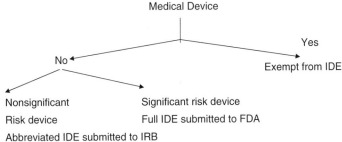

Figure 5.1 Significant and nonsignificant medical devices

- Form FDA 1571
- Investigational plan
- Investigator brochure
- Clinical protocols (study, investigator, facilities, IRB)
- Chemistry, manufacturing, control data
- Environmental impact statement
- Pharmacology and toxicology data
- Previous human experience
- Report of prior investigations
- Case report forms
- Risk analysis
- Description of the product
- Monitoring procedures
- Manufacturing information and environmental impact
- Investigator information
- Sales information
- Labeling
- Informed consent materials and IRB information

IDE Content

- Investigational plan
- Investigator brochure
- Clinical Protocols (study, investigator, facilities, IRB)
- Previous human experience
- Report of prior investigations
- Case report forms

- Risk analysis
- Description of the product
- Monitoring procedures
- Manufacturing information and environmental impact
- Investigator information
- Labeling
- Informed consent materials and IRB information

Marketing Applications   The following marketing applications exist for drugs and medical devices;

Drugs (part 314)

- New Drug Application (NDA)
- Supplemental NDA
- Abbreviated NDA—generics

Devices (part 814)

- Premarket approval application (PMA): Class III devices
- Supplemental PMA
- 510(K) premarket notification: Class II devices

Difference between 510(K) and PMA

- Volume information. Performance testing (i.e., bench, and in some cases animal) is often required and sufficient to address issues. Animal testing is required for almost all PMA submissions.
- Need for clinical data. Clinical data may be needed, depending on differences from predicate devices. Clinical data to demonstrate the safety and effectiveness of the device is required for all PMA submissions.
- Panel review. Panel review is not required for 510 k devices, but is required for the majority of PMA submission.
- Time to clearance or approval. In general, it takes 90 days for 510(K), and 180 days for PMA.
- Annual reporting requirements. This is not required for 510(K) devices but required for PMA devices

The classification of medical devices into classes I, II, and III is shown in Figure 5.2.

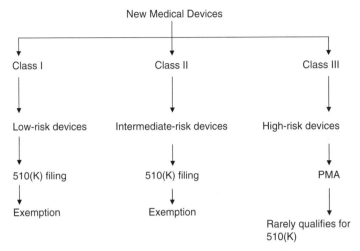

Figure 5.2 Classification of medical devices

510(K) Process

- File a 510(K) Notification of Intent to Market New Device (21 CFR 807).
- FDA determines *equivalence*.
- Clearance letter sent by FDA.
- FDA publishes decision and the summary on their website.

510(K) Requirements

- Statement of similarity. "A statement indicating the device is similar to and/or different from other products of comparable type in commercial distributions, accompanied by data to support the statement. This information may include an identification of similar products, materials, design consolidations, energy expected to be used or delivered by the device, and a description of the operational principles of the device."
- Additional information required by FDA 'for determining "substantial equivalence." May require more data on functional and scientific similarities.
- 510(K) summary must include:
    Sufficient detail to provide a basis for determination of "substantial equivalence" with a legally marketed product.
    "A description of the device explanation of how the device functions, the scientific concepts that form the basis for the device,

and the significant physical and performance characteristics of the device, such as device design, material used, and physical properties."

"A statement including a general description of the diseases or conditions that the device will diagnose, treat, prevent, cure, or mitigate if the indication statements are different from those of the legally marketed device an explanation as to why the differences are not critical to the intended therapeutic, diagnostic, prosthetic, or surgical use of the device, and why the differences do not affect the safety and effectiveness of the device when used as labeled."

"If the device has the same technological characteristics (i.e., design, material, chemical composition, energy source) as the predicate device a summary of the technological characteristics of the new device in comparison to those of the predicate device. If the device has different technological characteristics from the predicate device, a summary of how the technological characteristics of the device compare to a legally marketed device"

Substantial Equivalence   Substantial equivalence requires disclosure of the following:

- Similar products
- Similar materials
- Design consolidation
- Function
- Scientific concepts
- Design
- Characteristics
- Materials used
- Physical properties
- Diagnostic use and treatment
- Technological characteristics

The statement of substantial equivalence must then:

- Show differences are not critical.
- Show differences do not affect safety and effectiveness.
- Provide a comparison of the technological characteristics.

Off-label Use of Medical Devices   Manufacturers *can* disseminate credible scientific and medical information on off-label uses of devices to physicians. However, important to understand are the differences between:

- Making promotional claims for off-label uses.
- Disseminating truthful medical and scientific information to physicians about off-label uses.

The Practice of Medicine   The FDA is prohibited from interfering in the practice of medicine, but the FDA does regulate to keep a product sponsor from exerting influence on medical practice. Regulations require manufacturers to take action if they become aware of off-label use of their device:

- By providing adequate labeling (21 CFR 801.4).
- By meeting FDA expectations on permissible actions that are unclear.

It should be noted that making false or misleading statements in labeling constitutes misbranding prohibited under the Act (21 CFR 801.6). A new 510(K) claim is required to present a major change or modification in intended use [21 CFR 807.81(a)(3)]. A new 510(K) claim must be filed if an intended use differs from that of the legally marketed predicate device or exceeds the limitations of 510(K) exemptions (21 CFR 862–892.9).

Clinical Trial Design Differences

A fundamental difference between drug and device clinical studies is that a single confirmatory trial is required for devices. The standard for the regulatory approval of a pharmaceutical drug is to have two well-controlled phase III trials that demonstrate the safety and efficacy of the drug. Other differences between the clinical study design of drugs and devices may include the following:

- Feasibility and pivotal studies for devices versus phase I through III trials for drugs.
- Fewer subjects for device trials due to the large effect size. A typical pivotal device study includes 500 to 1000 subjects, whereas 1000 to 3000 subjects may participate in a pivotal drug study.

- Device trials may not be randomized or employ device features. The golden standard is a randomized study for both drugs and devices, but sometimes is difficult to adopt this design because of an ethical concern.
- Blinding/masking often is not possible with device studies.
- Device technology may change during a study.

A great deal of similarities exist between drugs and medical devices regarding the sponsor's responsibilities, the selection of investigators and study monitors, the monitoring of investigations and reporting of adverse events, investigator responsibilities, and record retention.

Sponsor Responsibilities

Drugs (312.50–52)

- Select qualified investigators.
- Ensure proper monitoring.
- Transfer obligations to a CRO if necessary.

Devices (812.40) The sponsor responsibilities are the same as those of drug trials, but there is no language on "transfer of obligations" to a CRO.

Selecting Investigators

Drugs (312.53)

- Select investigators qualified by training and experience.
- Ship investigational product (IP) only to participating investigators.
- Obtain investigator information (CV, Form FDA 1572, financial).

Devices (812.43) The selection process is the same as that for drug investigators drug, but no 1572. The information on selecting investigators is also listed in the investigator agreement.

Selecting Monitors

Drugs (312.53d) Monitors are selected based on their training and experience in monitoring previous investigations.

Devices (812.43d)   The selection of monitors is the same as for a drug trial.

Monitoring Investigations

Drugs (312.56)

- If noncompliance is discovered, secure compliance or discontinue IP shipments, terminate participation, and dispose/return of IP.
- FDA (312.70) can disqualify clinical investigators.
- Discontinue investigations if IP presents an unreasonable risk.

Devices (812.46)   The same rules apply as for the drug trial. In addition:

- Don't retract a device if that will jeopardize a subject's life (e.g., explant).
- FDA (812.119) can disqualify clinical investigators.
- Terminated studies of a significant risk device can be resumed only after FDA and IRB approval.

Sponsor Reporting to FDA

Drugs

- Protocol amendments (312.30) and IND amendments (312.31).
- IND safety reports of serious and unexpected drug-related adverse events (312.32).
- IND annual reports (312.33).
- New investigator Reports as part of protocol amendments.

Devices

- IDE supplemental applications (812.35).
- IDE safety reports of serious and unanticipated adverse device effects—UADE (812.150b).
- Annual progress reports and a final report, if a significant risk device is used (812.150b).
- Current investigator list every six months.
- Significant risk determination by IRB.

- Any sponsor request for device return, repair, or disposition (e.g., recall).
- Withdrawal of IRB approval.

Unanticipated Device Adverse Effect The serious adverse effect would be on health or safety or be any life-threatening problem or death caused by, or associated with a device. To be unanticipated, that effect, problem, or death would not have been previously identified in nature, severity, or degree of incidence in the investigational plan or application, or as any other unanticipated serious problem associated with a device that relates to the rights, safety, or welfare of patients.

Sponsor Record Retention

Drugs (312.57)

- Maintain investigator records, including financial disclosure.
- Maintain records of IP shipment/disposition.
- Retain records for two years after market approval or investigational use is discontinued.

Devices (812.140)

- *Same as for drug trial but*
- Retain records for two years after the information is no longer needed to support a market approval application.

Investigator Responsibilities

Drugs (312.60)

- Ensure that investigation was conducted according to investigational plan and followed FDA regulations.
- Protect rights, safety, welfare of subjects.
- Ensure that informed consent was obtained per part 50.

Devices (812.100)

- *Same as for drug plus*
- Language needed on permitting *potential subject recruitment* (e.g., interest), but not consent, prior to IRB and FDA approval (812.110).

Special Device and Drug Challenges Issues

Obtaining Informed Consent

1. Timing of informed consent can be difficult as subjects often enroll on same day of treatment (nonelective patient enrollment).
2. Indications for use of specific device may not be confirmed until sometime during a surgical procedure.
3. Subjects may require premedication for treatment.
4. Investigator skill and training with equipment varies.
5. Investigator training on device use may be difficult due to influx of new residents and fellows and rapid changes in technology.

Device Accountability

1. Monitoring and controlling device inventory may be difficult due to storage location (i.e., OR supply room) and device size/portability.
2. Some devices require "multiple-use" accountability.
3. Changes in device technology during trial may require frequent inventory changes.

Drug/Device Administration

Drugs (312.61)

- Administer IP to subjects under personal supervision or supervision of subinvestigator.
- Supply IP only to authorized persons.

Devices (812.110c)   The same rules apply as for the drug trial.

- Permit device to be used with subjects under investigator's supervision.
- There is no language about delegation to others.

Records Inspection by FDA

Drugs (312.58, 68)

- Sponsors and investigators will permit FDA to access, copy, and verify all records related to clinical investigations.
- Investigator records may identify subjects if FDA finds necessary.

Devices (812.145)   The same rules apply as for the drug trial.

FDA Websites on This Subject

Device Advice (CDRH). www.fda.gov/cdrh/devadvice/ide/index. shtml.

Investigational Device Exemptions Manual. www.fda.gov/cdrh/ manual/idemanul.html.

Good Clinical Practice (FDA). www.fda.gov/oc/gcp/default.htm.

BIMO Inspection Manuals (See IRB, Sponsors, or Investigators). www.fda.gov/ora/compliance_ref/bimo/default.htm.

COMBINATION PRODUCTS

Combination products combine a drug or biologic with a device. Examples of these products include drug-eluting stents, drug delivery systems, hemostatic sealants, photodynamic therapy, gene therapy, and other such investigational treatments. Combination products are subjected to FDA review by a combined team of medical device and drug product reviewers at the FDA.

The key challenging issue for a combination product is that the sponsor should be aware of the different clinical and scientific approaches at the FDA Center for Devices and Radiological Health (CDRH) compared with those at the Center for Drug Evaluation and Research (CDER). The determination of whether the combination product is a device, drug, or biologic by the FDA is determined mainly by the primary mode of action of the product. The following are examples of combination products that were determined to be devices, drugs, or biologics in accordance with the mode of action of the product:

Device. Drug-eluting stents, insulin pump, transdermal drug delivery patch, implantable drug delivery, pulmonary drug delivery, and photodynamic therapy.

Drug. Liposome plus chemotherapy, and AIDS protease inhibitor combination therapy.

Biologic. Collagen plus antiproliferative agent.

It should be noted that device designations are made by CDRH, drugs by CDER, and biologics by CBER. In most cases the same center will have the lead review and jurisdictional responsibility. Because of the growing number of combination products, the FDA has established the Office of Combination Products (OCP) to provide guidance to manufacturers pursuing development and market approval for combination products, and resolving jurisdictional and other issues that often arise during premarket review of combination products.

Combination Product Challenge

Many drug/device combination products are developed by device companies.

- A new drug delivery device, for example, may be designed to deliver an approved drug but with possibly different indications, mode of delivery, and drug dosage schedule.
- Without drug company authorization of access to its NDA and clinical/preclinical files, the device company may not be able to gain approval of its device to deliver a modified drug.

The drug-eluting stent paradigm could be a new trend.

The Office of Combined Product (OCP) and the FDA would then build on this novel approach to provide combination product regulation as follows:

- Incorporate drug labeling in the device IFU.
- Continue monitoring of the drug's adverse events by the device companies.
- Initiate a product-specific CDER/CBRH working group.

If the primary mode of action standard should be replaced, the primary jurisdiction would be assigned based on:

- The innovative drive in the combination.
- How the product will be used.
- Who will use the product.
- Which center has the real expertise in the medical/scientific area.

Because regulatory and jurisdictional issues are evaluated at the product development stage, *develop your strategy early*:

- Communicate with FDA early and often.
- Do not wait until the initiation of clinical studies to determine how FDA will regulate the combination.

- Do not hesitate to discuss the jurisdictional issues informally with the center's jurisdiction officers.
- Make sure your own company has the multidisciplinary expertise for the combination.
- Evaluate whether it is better to seek CDRH primary jurisdiction as opposed to CBER or CDER jurisdiction.
- Evaluate known precedents in judging whether CDRH jurisdiction would be more beneficial compared with CDER/CBER jurisdiction.
- Evaluate GMP/QSR issues for the combination, and propose a GMP jurisdictional strategy for the FDA at a pre-IND or pre-IDE meeting.

FDA Approval Process

The FDA approval of a combination product depends on the individual regulatory process of the drug and device components. A previous approval of the drug, even if approved for a different indication, makes it easier for approval than introducing an investigational drug. For an investigational drug, CDER has to be satisfied regarding the safety of the drug. Drug-eluting stents provide a clear example of this process. The Taxus coronary stent manufactured by Boston Scientific Corporation includes paclitaxel as the drug moiety in the combination product. This drug was approved earlier as an anticancer agent, so its approval facilitated the approval of the combination product because drug safety was established.

The main challenge to combination products is to define the primary mode of action (PMOA). It should be realized that some products don't have a clearly identifiable PMOA: no application specifically for combination products, and regulatory pathways sometimes not evident (e.g., need for cross labeling).

It is recommended that the sponsor request a pre-IDE/IND meeting from the FDA to discuss the proposed indication, potential benefit of the combination product, proposed FDA jurisdiction, preclinical testing, animal testing, and the proposed investigational plan for the clinical trial.

General Challenges of Combination Products

- No regulatory scheme designed specifically for combination products.

- No marketing application designed for combination products.
- The FDA work within existing statutory framework.

FDA–SPONSOR MEETINGS

FDA Meetings with Study Sponsors

The FDA encourages different type of clinical study meetings with the industry sponsors of these studies. These meetings often provide the following practical benefits to both the sponsors and the FDA:

1. Expedite review and approval of design testing and development plans.
2. Save money and time.
3. Allow for more collaborative approach between the FDA and the sponsor.
4. Minimize surprises.

It is recommended that before meeting with the FDA, sponsors should think carefully about the desired outcome and whether they are well-prepared for the meeting. There are several other issues that sponsors need to prepare prior to conducting these meetings: they should be prepared to manage their time effectively, bring qualified people to discuss focused questions, and never hesitate to ask for clarification. It should be also noted that if changes to device or protocol occur after the pre-IDE package was submitted, the meeting could be canceled or postponed. Sponsors should realize that guarantees or binding commitments do not result from these meetings, unless the meeting is intended to be a determination or agreement meeting. Studies or devices do not get approved at these meetings.

Timing of Meetings

Meetings may be held at any point in the *premarket phase*:

- Prior to conducting "proof-of-concept" animal studies.
- During the preclinical period.
- Prior to expanding clinical trials from feasibility to pivotal phase.
- Before the PMA submission.
- During the PMA submission.

- Following a postdeficiency letter for 510(K) or PMA.
- As an appeal after a final decision on a PMA or 510(K), or an IDE disapproval.
- As an agreement or determination meeting.

BIMO INSPECTION

The bioresearch monitoring (BIMO) program is an FDA program of on-site inspections for GCP and GLP. The program includes inspections of:

- Clinical Investigators
- Sponsors, monitors, CROs
- Institutional review boards
- Bioequivalence laboratories and facilities
- GLP facilities (nonclinical studies)

The program's objective is to verify the quality and integrity of bioresearch data, and to protect the rights and welfare of human research subjects. Study-specific data audits are announced in advance. Inspection includes interview with clinical investigator and an in-depth data audit to validate study findings and verify investigator compliance with regulations.

The BIMO inspection is based on the following written procedures

- Good Laboratory Practice
- Clinical Investigator
- Institutional Review Board
- Sponsor, CRO Monitors
- In vivo Bioequivalence

These documents can be obtained from http://www.fda.gov/oc/gcp/compliance.html.

Clinical Investigator Program

This inspection audits investigators conducting clinical trials of human and veterinary drugs, medical devices, and biologicals. Regulations that govern the responsibilities of investigators are found in:

- 21 CFR 312 (human drugs)
- 21 CFR 812 (medical devices)

GCP "BIMO" Inspections

BIMO inspections are performed for every new drug application and PMA. Additional BIMO inspections may be assigned based on complaints received by the FDA (from subjects, IRBs, or industry).

Compliance Classifications

- No action indicated. No objectionable conditions or practices were found during the inspection (or the objectionable conditions found do not justify further regulatory action).
- voluntary action indicated. Objectionable conditions or practices were found, but FDA is not prepared to take or recommend any administrative or regulatory action.
- Official action indicated:
    Regulatory and/or administrative actions will be recommended due to significant objectionable observations.
    Warning letters are sent and follow-up correspondence.

A follow-up with the FDA official action could lead to the rejection of the study or disqualification of the investigator.

Recommendations for Preparing Sponsor Site for BIOMO Inspection

- A qualified clinical or regulatory person from the sponsor site should meet the FDA inspectors. This person should have the capability of providing the FDA with the request in a timely manner.
- It is important to be positive and defend things when you have a supportive process; be ready to admit mistakes if any happened.
- The sponsor site should have readily available information about:
    Clinical personnel and their training records (personnel CVS, job descriptions, organizational charts).
    Investigators and clinical sites (information on study sites, information on important issues at study sites)

> Study data documents (CRFs, safety and effectiveness data, device accountability, monitoring reports, etc.)
>
> Procedures used in the study (clinical SOPs, any special procedures)

- The sponsor should be ready to answer any questions about the study data or procedures followed in the study.
- The clinical team (clinical scientists, biostatistician, etc.) who analyzed or put the data together should be ready for any FDA questions about the data.
- The clinical team who monitored the study should be ready for any FDA questions about the monitoring of the study.
- Responses to FDA inspectors should be provided accurately and documents provided in a timely manner.
- Good documentation and knowledge of the location of documents are critical to the success of the BIMO inspection.
- Data at study sites should be a mirror image of data at the sponsor site with all queries resolved and documented.
- During the course of the study be aware of and correct any deficiencies that were cited previously by the FDA such as:

  > Failure to adequately monitor the study.
  >
  > Failure to document monitoring visits.
  >
  > Failure to have clinical SOPs.
  >
  > Failure to maintain product accountability records.
  >
  > Failure to select qualified investigators.

INVESTIGATOR-INITIATED CLINICAL TRIALS

The classification of clinical studies into industry and investigator initiated trials is shown in Figure 5.3.

Sponsor Regulatory Requirements

- CV of principal and co-investigators (PI and CO-PI).
- Current medical licenses of participating physicians.
- 1572 Form (for drug studies).
- Lab normal values.
- Delegation of authority logs.

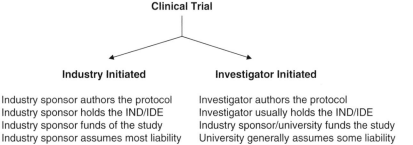

Figure 5.3 Clinical studies initiated by investigator and industry

- IRB approval.
- FDA approval.

Budgeting: Key Budget Items at Study Site

The review by the study site of the study budget can take a long time to finalize, a task that must be completed in order to sign off the research contract. To cut down the review time, the sponsor of the study is encouraged to finalize and provide budget that includes the following items:

- Up-front administrative costs
- Institutional review board fee
- Research pharmacy costs (for drug studies)
- Pharmacy setup fee (for drug studies)
- Ongoing drug dispensing costs (for drug studies)
- Study initiation costs
- Patient recruitment costs
- Screening efforts (and cost of screen failures)
- Patient enrollment costs
- Patient care/services
- Hospital/outpatient services (e.g., cath lab, diagnostic services, radiology lab, nursing)
- Professional fees for other physicians' services
- Investigator effort
- Compensation for managing the study
- Professional fees

- Research staff compensation and other personnel costs
- Facilities and equipment
- Supplies
- Travel (investigator meetings/conferences)
- Subject payments
- Record retention costs
- Overhead/indirect costs
- Miscellaneous (e.g., phone, fax, shipping costs)

Final Documents Required for Contract Sign-Off

The following documents will need a final sign-off at the study sites:

- Final Protocol
- Final Budget
- Financial Disclosure Forms
- IRB Approval
- Investigator Exception Letter

In investigator-initiated clinical trials the following questions should be answered precisely:

- Who are the parties? Usually the studies include a partnership between an industrial company who makes the product and an academic institution who is interested in conducting and executing the study.
- What are their roles? The responsibilities of each party should be detailed in the research contract between the parties. Usually the industrial company provides the research product and the academic group conducts, executes, and manages the study.
- How can you manage the risk of investigator initiated research?

Industry

- Ineffective use of resources (financial and personnel) that do not support the strategic plan.
- Lack of up-front planning leading to potential nonvalidated data that cannot be utilized for publication or support of FDA submission.
- Data results oppose current data results or strategic plan.

- Inappropriate budgets suggesting marketing influence.
- Legal issues arising from noncompliance.

Institution/Investigator

- Local sponsorship ambiguity.
- Inadequate resources to act as sponsor.
- Presentation/publication of nonvalidated data (false claims).
- Pivotal impact for research subject safety.
- Legal issues from noncompliance to regulation.
- Lack of indemnification of site from funding sources.

What are the criteria for an appropriate investigator initiated research project? How should investigator initiated research be reviewed and processed?

The party who is responsible for planning and executing the study prepares the clinical protocol, monitoring plan, and so forth. After review by the involved parties, the research is reviewed by the FDA and the IRB.

CHAPTER 6

Challenges of Global Clinical Studies and the CE Mark Process

The critical issue facing many medical device manufacturers today is how to bridge the gaps between FDA's regulation of the United States and the Medical Devices Directive (MDD) of the European Union. Underlying the complexities and the differences between the two systems are fundamental similarities. Most important, both systems have the same goals: to ensure that a medical device company produces a safe product and that the company can do so consistently. Both regimens stress good manufacturing and design control processes. Only companies that meet the MDD requirements receive a CE mark, which allows their products to be sold in the EU market.

Even for companies that have satisfied FDA premarket approval requirements, the MDD requirements can be complex. Conformity assessment, the processes and procedures by which companies demonstrate that their products meet CE marking requirements, varies depending on the class of product; therefore closing the gaps between the US and the EU requirements can vary according to product type. It should be noted that in the EU there are four classes (class I, class IIa, class IIb, and class III), while FDA has three (class I, class II, and class III).

The Design and Management of Medical Device Clinical Trials: Strategies and Challenges, by Salah Abdel-aleem
Copyright © 2010 John Wiley & Sons, Inc.

Furthermore, in the United States, submissions for products in the same class have historically had different requirements for premarket notification—510(K) as compared with premarket approval (PMA)—whereas EU product approval submissions are based solely on class, and each submission must meet exactly the same requirements.

The FDA has increased the range of information it requires to include technical and safety standards, risk analysis, and design control, and the scope of a comprehensive 510(K). FDA deals with many of the same questions as the essential requirements and covers the same ground regarding inspections. As a result companies that have recently developed comprehensive 510(K)s and PMA applications should meet most EU requirements. Many of the ISO or other standards required by FDA are either the same as or equivalent to EU harmonized standards; therefore, if a company can meet FDA requirements, it is often approved by the EU standards.

This chapter casts light onto the importance and increased number of global clinical trials, and also the FDA recommendations for accepting foreign clinical sites in global studies. Operational tips and recommendations are provided to consolidate the gaps between the US and EU clinical regulations, and also clinical practices. An introduction to the CE mark and its requirement is therefore presented, along with the important difference between the CE mark and market clearance by the FDA regarding the classification of medical devices and the device clearance process. Device clearance in the EU depends on demonstrating the safety of the device and the performance (that it performs as intended). The performance measurements could be technical measurements that relate to the subject and device. For example, the technical success of stents, or the technical success in vessel diameter methods before or after the intervention, could be representative of the performance of the device. In contrast, the approval process in the United States is dependent on demonstrating the safety and effectiveness of the device. The effectiveness of the device means the clinical utility of the device or surrogate measurements that are directly related to the clinical benefits. Given the last example of stents, an effectiveness endpoint could reflect the clinical utility of the stent system such as reduction of major adverse events in terms of mortality, cardiac infarction, and stroke.

GLOBAL TRIAL CONSIDERATIONS

There is tremendous pressure on drug and device sponsors to increase the involvement of international clinical sites as a part of global clinical trials for the following reasons:

- The increase of the sample size and need to enroll more subjects into the trial in a timely fashion. International sites may offer large subject populations with the same characteristics of the disease or condition.
- The availability of specific subject populations with certain conditions in foreign countries such as infectious, bacterial, and viral diseases.
- The reduction of the cost of conducting these trials in some foreign countries:

    Lower cost for medications, investigators, and hospitalization in some countries.

    Cheaper supportive administration cost for the trial.
- Fewer competitor trials at international sites which will speed enrollment.
- High growth market in the region in the future.

However, several challenges of operating global clinical trials may exist:

- Lack of harmonized standards.
- Varying regulatory regimens/timelines.
- Data protection/privacy.
- Informed consent (language, culture, and geopolitical barriers).
- Trial participation rates.
- Investigators/workforce.

The main benefits for patients, investigators, and countries in conducting global clinical trials in emerging countries are:

- Participants enjoy improved care.
- Training of resources is in accord with high international standards.
- Standards of medical practice are improving.

Current Situation in Europe

The expansion of the European Union has led to inconsistencies in European research ethics. It is important, however, for all of Europe to harmonize ethical standards of researchers. Failure to understand these differences could compromise and bias the results of clinical trials, and their interpretations. The challenge is to discern variations in local, national, and international customs and practice, while developing new ways of discovering and understanding the emerging ethical and legal issues for clinical trials in Europe today.

Regional Ethical Issues

Regional ethical considerations include important issues like disregard of ethics in a region, which would have an effect on the design, conduct, and analysis of clinical trials. Informed consent issues may include: How is the informed consent perceived by patients, physicians (medical personnel), and researchers in general? How is the principle of informed consent being implemented in these countries for clinical trials? How could the practice of informed consent be improved in the region? Ethical standard issues may include: How are (international/EU) ethical standards implemented in clinical trials? How could EU standards improve the ethical quality of clinical trials in new member and candidate states? Ethics committees considerations may include questions about the current role of ethics committees: How is the responsibility to the community of ethics committee members perceived in the region? How could their role be improved? How may the standards of ethics committees and procedures be improved? The composition of ethics committees varies greatly among EU member states. Some are knowledgable and demonstrate independence; others lack both knowledge and independence. Standardized ethics forms, processes, and documentation are needed within the member states, and throughout the European Union, in order to make the ethics application process less bureaucratic and more uniform and effective.

Conflict of interest issues may include: How is conflict of interests perceived (e.g., social acceptance) and regulated in the region? Are conflicts of interests increasing/decreasing/remaining the same? Does the availability of provision of healthcare in the region and the type of provision such as private, state, or insurance-based affect the design, conduct, and analysis of clinical trials or affect medical research? Do the hospitals support research and clinical trials, for example, by providing insurance protection "indemnity," time, peer review, statistical advice, and a research friendly atmosphere? Are patients in the country generally willing to take part in clinical trials/medical research and why? Does this vary with different types of research or the type and severity of illness or the age and sex of the patient? Are there any traditional or established medical or clinical practices or clinical organizational issues that affect the design, conduct, and analysis of clinical trials or research? How has European law and its local national implementation affected the design conduct and analysis of clinical trials and research?

Research is becoming disproportionately bureaucratic in some states:

- Where research is discouraged, the success of some legitimate projects may be impeded and divert effort away from good project design.
- Researchers detered from taking part in clinical research may be likely to carry out animal or molecular research, where productivity is greater as bureaucracy is less.
- Commercial research, by pharmaceutical companies, is predominately taking place in new member states.
- With the decline in funding, time, support, and facilities for independent scientific research, hospital support for independent scientific research is declining, and focused on cost versus patient turnover. Private medicine is taking a greater hold on health care, but in this sector research is virtually absent.

Cultural Issues

Are there any specific cultural influences in the country that have an effect on the design, conduct, and analysis of clinical trials? In some EU countries there is implicit trust of patients in their doctors. This results in relatively high patient compliance for clinical trials. Also cultural aspects are often associated with religious traditions. More work is needed to be done for a deeper understanding of cultural influences on the practice of clinical trials in Europe.

It is hard to cover the differences between countries in just a few questions. Research involving a greater number of countries is needed. Such research should be quantitative as well as qualitative. It should be noted that the impact of globalization on culture cannot be ignored:

- How much do the patients in the country agree with medical experiment on them? It was found in some countries that people are more cautious with medical experimentation on close ones, than on themselves.
- How much are people willing to accept medical experiment on sick persons: themselves, relatives, or close friends? How does the press (in the country), the media react generally, to experiments made by human beings? The press can be distrustful of human experimentation, sometimes with good reason. Scientists are used to the concepts of uncertainty and debate. However, this does not fit well with sound journalism. Scientists need to be more aware of the limitations

of the press and the need to prepare media-friendly statements. Such statements should not overdramatize findings and should be communicated in language that is clear to the nonexpert.

- Do doctors easily recommend medicines and techniques insufficiently known, or with uncertain results? Doctors are usually wary of recommending medicines and techniques that are insufficiently known or that have uncertain side effects on patients.

Technology Issues

Are there any technological influences specific to a country that may have an effect on the design, conduct, and analysis of clinical trials? Do new medical technologies go through a controlled clinical trial process before general use in your country? Is ethical approval obtained before the use of newly designed medical equipment on patients? Is there any exemption for locally (university or hospital) designed equipment (as opposed to that produced by a large manufacturer)? Are there any local (government or charitable agencies) grants available for the development of new medical equipment?

GLOBAL HARMONIZATION TASK FORCE CHALLENGES

Challenges to Task Force

The challenges the global harmonization task force faces could be summarized as follows:

- Regulatory paradigms differ from one country to the other.
- Maturity of systems varies.
- Significant cultural differences present among European countries.
- Nonbinding "guidance" into legislation and/or regulation are difficult to incorporate even for FDA in short time period.
- Economic incentives and disincentives.

Challenges to Consent Seeking in Clinical Trials

Additional challenges pertain to poor handling of:

- Informed consent
- Confidentiality

- Conflict of Interest
- Standard of care
- Lack of honest reporting of data
- Misconduct and professional incompetence of researchers
- Clearly defined benefits to the research host community

FDA RECOMMENDATIONS ON ACCEPTANCE OF FOREIGN CLINICAL SITES

The basic recommendations of the US Department of Health and Human Services to the FDA when international sites are proposed are:

1. Institutional review board must adhere to international ethical standards, the Declaration of Helsinki, or the International Conference on Harmonization, as well as the local regulations.
2. Qualified investigators must be subject to frequent monitoring and FDA inspections.
3. The international site must be an adequate research facility.

The specific recommendations of the US Department of Health and Human Services to the FDA when internal sites are proposed for foreign countries are:

1. Obtain more information about the performance of foreign institutional review boards, since in many foreign countries the FDA has minimal information about the operating IRBs.
2. Help foreign boards build capacity by working with the US Department of Health or other government agencies (e.g., NIH).
3. Encourage sponsors to obtain attestations from foreign investigators that they adhere to the principals of research.
4. Encourage greater sponsor monitoring.
5. Develop a database to track the growth and location of foreign research.

OPERATIONAL TIPS ON CONDUCTANCE OF GLOBAL CLINICAL TRIALS

Certain operational procedures are important in global clinical studies as international sites are planned to be included in the study and also the final clinical report as would be submitted to the FDA as well as other international regulatory bodies. First off, early communication is encouraged between the US and international clinical teams to harmonize some of the regulations and the procedures of the study protocol to make foreign regulations compatible with those of the United States. Examples of the harmonization may be in the area of reporting of units of measurements in the CRFs, reporting of adverse events, or the use of concomitant medications.

Differences may exist between the US and certain international sites in the reporting time periods of serious adverse events from the investigator to the sponsor or to regulatory authority. The US regulations and the EU standard differ in their definition, or wording, regarding the seriousness or severity of an adverse event. The EU regulations (EN 540) address adverse event seriousness based on the adverse event severity grading (mild, moderate, severe, and life threatening). The standard explains that a severe adverse event satisfies almost the same condition listed for a serious adverse event in an IDE study (causes death, hospitalization, or prolonged hospitalization; requires intervention; results in a congenital anomaly, malignancy, or residual damage). The IDE regulations of the United States use the term *serious* as defined above. To avoid differences in the definition of the seriousness of adverse events, sponsors try to define adverse events based on seriousness as well as severity.

So, to avoid confusion about the units of measurements between the US and international sites, alternatives for unit definitions may be provided, or clinical sites may be instructed on which units that they should use in the study. Another example of synchronization of the clinical protocol procedures in global clinical trials is the use of protocol concomitant medications. Certain international sites use other alternative drugs than those used in the United States due to economic or other reasons. To avoid having numerous protocol deviations, the option of these alternative medications should be provided in the study protocol if it has no effect on the study outcome (for more details on the global clinical studies, see Chapter 8).

Furthermore US and international clinical teams should harmonize CRFs and provide multiple alternatives for unit definitions, or instruct investigators on which units to specifically use to avoid any confusion over these units. Because of the use of different units in Europe as compared to the United States either both unit definitions and conversion should be given to the site or the sites should be instructed to use specific units. For example, the units of items such as weight (should be defined in lbs or kgm), height (in or cm), blood glucose (mg/dl or mM), and also if these parameters are defined by a single unit system. It is important to reconcile as well differences in the definition of certain adverse events and their reporting timelines between the US and other international regions.

Finally, in device trials, center-to-center variations in device effects can result from physician experience or training in using or implanting the device. Other variations may be due to differing patient populations, patient management systems, and reporting practices. A scientifically credible explanation is required to account for variation of data across study centers. Comparative analysis may be further critical when a multicenter trial includes international sites to take note of any differences among the international sites in the quality of their health systems.

Challenge of Clinical Trial Distribution

According to one of the most significant factors affecting the potency of medicinal agents is the ability to maintain them in controlled environments.

Distribution Risks

Temperature excursions during the storage, handling, or distribution of temperature-sensitive clinical trial material pose significant safety and financial risks:

Key Risks

- Compliance must be with global regulatory and standards-based requirements.
- Patient is administered as an unsafe product.
- Product is rejected.
- Inconsistency occurs within batches.

Regulatory Trends

- Responsibility for the product distribution ultimately resides with the manufacturer, but accountability is shared across the supply chain.
- Increased oversight, management, and control of environmental conditions must be provided across the entire supply chain.

- Temperature control and monitoring have increased importance.
- Patient safety is given, heightened priority with the focus being on product quality.

CE MARK PROCESS AND CHALLENGES

The CE mark is derived from the French abbreviation "Conformité Européene." The CE is a mandatory design review and risk identification and mitigation process that attempts to minimize product risks to humans, animals, and the environment. The CE mark is required for selling products to and within over 29 European countries. It proves to the buyer—or user—that the product fulfills all essential safety and environmental requirements as these are defined in the European Directives. The CE mark directive (93/68/EEC) was adopted in 1993.

The CE marking is adopted by member countries of the European Union, namely Austria, Belgium, Cyprus, the Czech Republic, Denmark, Estonia, Finland, France, Germany, Greece, Hungary, Ireland, Italy, Latvia, Lithuania, Luxembourg, Malta, the Netherlands, Poland, Portugal, Slovakia, Slovenia, Spain, Sweden, and the United Kingdom. Countries of the European Free Trade Area (EFTA) and European Economic area (EEA)—namely Iceland, Norway, Liechtenstein, and Switzerland—also honor the CE mark. Future participation countries may include Bulgaria, Romania, and Turkey. The CE mark is sufficient to allow exporting of drugs and medical devices to all EC members.

CE Marking Process

To comply with the CE mark requirements:

1. Identify the applicable EU/CE Directive(s). Multiple directives may cover a single product, so the applicable directives that cover essential requirement of the product must be identified.
2. Assess your product to the "essential requirements." Products must meet the essential requirements that are applicable in the directives to protect people, animals, and the environment.
3. Choose appropriate conformity assessment module. CE conformity assessment is divided into a modular system and procedure manufactures must be completed to prove that their product.
4. If required, select a notified body. Your conformity assessment module will indicate if you need to hire the services of a notified

body (NOBO). A NOBO must be located within the geographical bounds of the European Union. An approval by a NOBO located anywhere in the European Union is valid throughout Europe. Consider using US affiliates of European NOBOs.

5. Apply relevant product standards. Examples are the International Organization for Standardization (ISO) and the European Standard (EN).

6. Conduct any required testing. Some standards require product testing. So select a laboratory that is familiar with the product and test, and choose a test laboratory notified body.

7. Assemble and submit all necessary documentation. The key documents are the Technical File (TF), Declaration of Conformity, and the CE marking logo.

8. Appoint an authorized representative. If required, appoint an authorized representative, which may be a person or an organization that ensures that a manufacturer's technical file is made readily available in Europe, and acts on your behalf in the event of a challenge or audit. This requirement is mandatory for medical devices.

9. Address European recycling and disposition requirements.

10. Affix the CE marking logo.

CE Marking and European Harmonization

The European Union developed CE marking to sanction product safety and health concerns in the trade of drugs and medical devices within Europe. Before CE marking, manufacturers had to comply with multiple, and often inconsistent, national product compliance systems. The CE marking is managed by Directorate General Enterprise, a body in the European Commission. The European Commission is the approximately equivalent to cabinet agencies in the United States. CE marking cover a wide range of activities pertaining to the design, development, production, documentation, sale, and distribution of a product. Manufacturers must review, and even alter, a product to ensure its compliance with the CE mark in design, performance, materials, labeling, documentation, manufacturing process, and packaging. Under EU law, the company that "places a product on the market or into service" is responsible for the CE marking. The sponsor of the product may be a manufacturer, distributor, agent, or representative, for example. However most often the physical manufacturer is ultimately responsible for the CE marking. The benefits of the CE mark can be summarized as follows: it offers a wide market of 455 million people, which is comparable to the US market. The CE steps may result in a safer product and/or an enhanced manufacturing process, but also CE marking has simplified for manufactures the need to comply with multiple conflicting national compliance systems.

CE marking is enforced at a national level by customs officials, market surveillance authorities, and the courts. Noncompliant products may be pulled out of service and permanently banned from European markets. Manufacturers and suppliers violating CE marking requirements may even incur criminal and/or civil penalties.

CE Marking Procedure

1. Make a certification inquiry/request for proposal.
2. Submit an application form/registration.
3. Identify the directive standard.
4. Review the technical file.
5. Comply with the audit/inspection and testing.
6. Make a CE notification/national laboratory.
7. Obtain verification/declaration of conformity/affix CE mark.
8. Receive a certificate of compliance/verification.
9. Submit to a surveillance audit.
10. Market to a satisfied customer.

A Harmonizing Challenge

Different areas of government oversee different policy areas for clinical studies, making it difficult to staff one GHTF/ISO group to address all issues. A Global Harmonization Task Force (GHTF) coordinates regulations.

INTERNATIONAL STANDARD ISO 14155

The International Standard ISO 14155 has the following purposes:

- Applied to assess clinical performance of medical devices in human subjects.
- Specifies the requirements for the conduct of clinical investigation to determine the performance and safety of medical devices in human subjects.

- Provides the framework for written procedures for the design, implementation, data collection, documentation, and the conduct of the clinical investigation.
- ISO 14155-1 defines procedures for the conduct and performance of clinical investigation of medical devices to protect human subject, ensure the scientific conduct of the investigation, and to assist sponsors, monitors, investigators, ethics committees, regulatory authorities, and other bodies involved in conformity assessments of medical devices.
- ISO 14155-2 provides requirements for the preparation of a clinical investigation plan (CIP) of medical devices.

ISO 14155-1

Scope   ISO 14155-1 is applicable to all clinical investigations:

- Pre-CE mark investigations
- Postmarket surveillance
- Marketing studies

This international standard defines procedures for the conduct and performance of clinical investigations of medical devices. It specifies general requirements pertains to:

- all clinical investigations of medical devices whose clinical performance and safety is being assessed in human subjects.
- specifies requirements for the organization, conduct, monitoring, data collection and documentation of the clinical investigation of a medical device

Adverse Event Definitions   The New wording on adverse events introduces the term "serious" instead of "severe" and "near serious adverse events" for two reasons:

- The terminology "serious" instead "severe" is more in conformity with ICH guidelines.
- The terminology "near serious" adverse device effect harmonizes better with MEDDEV (medical device) guidelines.

Serious adverse event is defined as:

- Death
- Serious deterioration in the health of the subject resulting in:

  Life-threatening disease or injury.

  Permanent impairment of a body structure or a body function.

  Inpatient hospitalization or prolongation of existing hospitalization.

  Medical or surgical intervention to prevent permanent impairment to body structure or a body function.

ISO 14155-1 and MEDDEV Compared

- MEDDEV does not mention inpatient hospitalization or prolongation of existing hospitalization.
- MEDDEV includes incidents affecting the health of clinical staff, whereas ISO does not mention these persons.

ISO 14155-1 and .FDA Definitions ISO 14155 and FDA have similar definitions of severe adverse events. However, a serious adverse device effect is defined in ISO 14155-1 as:

> Adverse device effect that resulted in any of the consequences characteristics of a serious adverse event or that might have led to any of these consequences if suitable action had not been taken or intervention had not be made or if circumstances had been less opportune.

A serious adverse device effect in MEDDEV is defined as a reportable incident: "those which led to a death, those which led to a serious deterioration in the state of health of a patient, user or other person." Note that ISO 14155 does not mention "user or other person."

The serious adverse device effect in the second part of the MEDDEV definition introduces the terminology "near serious incident." Compare this with the FDA definition:

> Unanticipated adverse device effect is any serious adverse effect on health or safety, any life-threatening problem or death caused by, or associated iwth a device, if that effect, problem or death was not previously identified in nature, severity, or degree of incidence in application; or any other unanticipated problem associated with a device that relates to the rights, safety, or welfare of subjects.

How to Implement ISO and MEDDEV Procedures?

- In clinical department, update the different definitions in SOPs, protocols, and other instructions (CRF instructions, etc.) with new ISO 14155 definitions.
- Overall vigilance of company procedures should make clear the distinctions between MEDDEV-related to CE-marked devices and ISO 14155 definitions for clinical investigations.

Additional Remarks   The timelines for reportable events are the same as those for CE-marked devices. Therefore continue to separate serious adverse events from near serious adverse events.

New Definitions   Note that these definitions provide only guidance; companies should continue to use definitions that are useful in the context of their practices.

- Coordinating clinical investigator. This category corresponds with the old EN 540 definition of principal investigator.
- Principal investigator. The new definition designates this as the center-specific principal investigator.
- Investigation center/site (absent in EN 540).
- Source data (absent in EN 540).
- Source documents (absent in EN 540).

Justification for a Clinical Investigation

- Introduces the need for a review of the published literature and available unpublished medical and scientific data and information. EN 540 only states that an investigator brochure is needed to provide a literature review. Note this would not necessarily be a type of justification for the clinical investigation.
- Balances residual risks against anticipated benefits of the clinical investigations.
- Mentions whether a required risk analysis is to be performed prior to conducting a clinical investigation.
- Indicates points in line with FDA guidance and also awareness of terms of EU and global trials.

General Requirements   Regulatory clearance needs to be obtained prior to starting a clinical investigation; this requirement is not mentioned in EN 540 but should be listed in the appropriate clinical SOPs. Further the privacy and confidentiality of information about each subject must be ensured in reports and any publication of data. Separate lists need to be maintained with the subject names identified. Note that:

EN 540: no mention of patient list.

21 CFR part 812: patient identification is required.

Data Protection Act and HIPAA: these are in contradiction on the use of patient names, initials, or date of birth. GCP regulators are currently looking into how to comply on these matters. The main concern is web-based data.

To assure the patient about confidentiality, the standard practice is to do this by informed consent and inform the patient as to:

· Which data are collected at which time points.
· Who processes the data, and requests access to source documents.
· Where are the data processed (in which country).
· Restricted access.
· Requests from national authorizations where applicable.

Suspension or early termination of a clinical investigation could come with new provisions. But this is incompletely indicated in EN 540 under the sponsor's obligations (reporting to the EC is not mentioned in EN 540).

Regarding document and data control:

· All documents and data are to be produced and maintained in such as way as to assure control of documents and data and to protect the subject's privacy as far as reasonably practical.
· The new section in EN 540 omits mention of this issue, but document and data control are in line with 21 CFR part 812.

The documentation should account for all subjects. Besides all subjects enrolled in the clinical investigation, those withdrawn from the investigation or lost to follow-up) should be accounted for and documented as well.

The new section reflects EN 540 and is in line with 21 CFR part 812.

On access to preclinical and clinical information, the monitor shall have access to the source documents and other information needed to ensure investigator compliance with the CIP, and applicable rules and regulations and to assess the progress of the Clinical investigation.

On the auditing of all clinical information, the new section also reflects EN 540, and is in line with 21 CFR part 812: "The clinical investigator shall allow auditing of their clinical investigation procedures."

Informed Consent   EN 540 decribes hardly any of the process and none of the contents of informed consent, whereas 21 CFR part 50 is very detailed with regards to informed consent. Both ISO 14155 and 21 CFR part 50 require a written informed consent compared to EN 540, which states "preferably in writing."

- Guidance on process for obtaining consent:
    Avoid coercion of or undue influence of subjects to participate.

    Do not waive or appear to waive subject's legal rights.

    Use nontechnical and understandable language.

    Provide ample time for subject to consider participation in study.

    Include dated signature of subject and investigator.

    Describe special circumstances.

    Process documented in the CIP (clinical investigator program).
- Guidance for content of informed consent and informed consent statement (nearly in line with 21 CFR.)
- Informed consent statement.
- Informed consent agreement:
    Must agree to participate in and comply with investigation.

    Must agree to his/her personal physician being informed of his/her participation or state his/her disagreement to the release of this information.

    Must agree to the use of his/her relevant personal data for the purpose of the clinical investigation.

Documentation

- Investigator brochure, which puts new emphasis on results of risk analyses.
- Other documents:
    CIP (clinical investigator program)

Current *signed and dated* CV of each investigator*
Names of participating institutions (investigator list)
Ethics committee opinions
Correspondence with authorities*
Agreements*
Insurance certificates*
Informed consent forms and other patient information
CRF
Forms for reporting Aes and ADE*
Names and contact addresses of monitors*

Sponsor's Responsabilities Sponsor's responsibilities are fully detailed as:

- Clinical investigation activities remain the responsibility of the sponsor even if some activities are subcontracted to a third party.
- All devices designated for use in the clinical investigation must be fully described.
- Deviations must be followed up by the sponsor and cleared.
- The sponsor communicates SAEs to other investigators based on perceived risk.
- The sponsor informs investigators of the developmental stages of a device and the clinical investigation requirements.
- The sponsor ensures that there is accurate device accountability with traceability of its applications.

Monitor's Responsibilities The monitor must verify that:

- Compliance exists with investigation plan.
- Device is used in compliance with the investigation plan.
- Data are accurate and accord with the source documents.
- Maintenance and calibration of equipment proceeds as planned.
- Withdrawals and noncompliance subjects are documented.

Investigator's Responsibilities

- Qualifications of the investigators are defined.
- Resources are adequate.

*Worded with totally new guidance compared to EN 540, but this is in line with the IDE requirements in the United States.

- Conflicts of interest are avoided.
- Subjects are well acquainted with clinical investigation plan before signing it.
- Support monitor performs source document verification and files correct case report forms.
- Ethics committees is informed about serious adverse device effects. Note that some ethics committees may want to be informed about all SAEs and not only those that are device related.
- Sponsor is informed about AEs and SAEs.
- Identification of Investigation is identified in medical records.
- Subjects have available emergency care.
- Accuracy, legibility, and security of all clinical data is ascertained both during and after the clinical investigation:

   All case report forms should be signed by support monitor.

   Any alterations are to be made by authorized personnel, initialed and dated with original entry retained for comparison.
- All data are retained.
- All devices are accounted for in the center. Note that the quantity of devices received should be reconciled with quantities used, discarded, or returned.

Annexes   Informative annexes have been included on:

- Ethics committee submission documents.
- Literature review.
- Final report writing.

Future of ISO 14155 Part 1

- Changes to be expected for some terminology and definitions of adverse events, protocol, and final report.
- Changes to be expected in design requirements of clinical investigations.
- Changes to harmonize the standard more in line with ICH.
- More explicit information on what constitutes an "audit," an "independent data monitoring committee," "device malfunction," and so forth.
- More explicit definition of "unforseeable risks" in informed consents.

ISO 14155 Part 2

Clinical investigations of medical devices for human subjects:

- Must present a clear identification of the clinical investigation plan.
- Must provide a list of all participating parties. Sponsor, Investigators, co-investigators, monitors, investigation centers, and other institutions.
- Must include monitoring arrangements and source document verification.
- CIP must specify data and quality management procedures.
- Must include synopsis, and approval and agreement section. Coordinating investigator and principal investigator in each center approves and signs the CIP.
- Must identify and describe the medical device:

    Competent authorities want to avoid major changes to the device during the clinical investigation as this can lead to invalid data merging.

    The purpose and contraindications of the device should be clear.

    All materials in contact with body fluids should be described.

    Use, preparation, handling requirements, and pre-use safety checks should be specified fully.

    The necessary training prior to use should be summarized.

    All necessary procedures involved in the use of the device should be described.
- Must include a literature review supporting the rationale for conducting the trial.
- Must review preclinical testing, existing clinical data, and device's risk analysis.
- Must present the objectives of the investigation.
- Must include in the design of the clinical investigation:

    Controls.

    Methods avoiding bias.

    Endpoints.

    Variables to be measured, and when.

    Test equipment to be used.

    Eligibility criteria.

    Definition of the point of enrollment.

    Description of procedures.

Criteria for withdrawal.

Number of subjects with statistical justification.

Adverse event recording, safety data analysis.

Duration of use of the device if applicable.

Any foreseeable factors that may potentially influence the results.

- Must include statistical considerations.

Justification of sample size. The standard is to justify consideration of small sample sizes for early pilot trials.

Pass/fail criteria.

Provisions for interim analyses.

Criteria for accounting of data and subgroup analyses.

Deviations of clinical investigation plan.

Need for reporting of investigator to sponsor, and if relevant to EC and CA.

- Must consider amendments to CIP.
- Must report AEs and SAEs.
- Must explain early termination of investigation.
- Must present a publication plan.
- Must fill case report forms.
- Must include an informative annex for guidance on the case report forms.

DIFFERENCES BETWEEN FDA AND CE MARK CLINICAL TRIALS

There is a major difference in the way that devices are regulated in the European Union compared with the United States, especially in the clinical data required for premarket approval. This has introduced significant differences in time-to-market approval for the United States compared with the European Union, particularly in the case of high-risk class III devices. The time needed to market a medical device in the European Union is shorter than in the United State.

EU Procedures

The vast majority of medical devices in the European Union from surgical gloves to life-sustaining implantable devices, such as heart valves, is regulated by the Medical Devices Directive (MDD). This means that medical devices bearing a CE marking can circulate freely throughout the European Union without any market barriers.

CE Marking Process

A key aspect of medical device regulation in the European Union is that the responsibility for ensuring that devices meet Essential Requirements lies with the manufacturer. The classification of medical devices is different from the FDA classification. In the United States medical devices are labeled as class I, II, or III. Class I are low-risk devices, class II are medium-risk devices, and class III are high-risk devices. In the European Union medical devices are labeled as class I, class IIa, class IIb, or class III. Class I are low-risk devices, class IIa medium risk devices, Class IIb high medium-risk devices, and class III are high-risk devices. For low-risk devices (class I) such as a tongue depressor or colostomy bag, the manufacturer is allowed to self-declare conformity with the Essential Requirements. For medium- to high-risk devices (class IIa, class IIb, or class III), the manufacturer must call on a third party to assess conformity. To some degree, the manufacturer may choose among methods for "conformity assessment" of the device and/ or manufacturing system. The end result is certificates of conformity that enable the manufacturer to apply a CE marking to the product.

Another major aspect of the CE marking process is that unlike pharmaceutical products, the medical device Conformity Assessment is not conducted by a regulatory agency for drugs and devices (a member state's Competent Authority or a central authority, e.g., the EMEA). The CE marking system relies heavily on Notified Bodies to implement regulatory control over medical devices.

The majority of Notified Bodies are independent commercial organizations that are designated, monitored, and audited by the relevant member states via the national Competent Authorities. Currently there are more than 50 active Notified Bodies within the European Union. A company is free to choose any Notified Body to cover the particular class of device under review. After approval, postmarket surveillance functions are the responsibility of a member state via the Competent Authority.

Clinical Data Requirements

What clinical data is required by the EU medical device regulations? How does this differ from FDA requirements of the United States? As previously mentioned, the need for clinical data in the CE marking process arises from the requirement to demonstrate that a device is safe, that it performs as intended by the manufacturer, and that any risks are acceptable when weighed against the benefits of the device. The term "clinical data" is a broad concept that includes everything from bench testing to clinical trials in human subjects. As stated in the MDD, the clinical data used for CE marking may be in one of two forms:

- A compilation of the relevant scientific literature currently available on the intended purpose of the device and the techniques employed, together with, if appropriate, a report containing a critical evaluation of the compilation.
- The results and conclusions of a specifically designed clinical investigation.

The first option, also referred to as the "literature route," is commonly used by manufacturers for the CE marking of low- to medium-risk devices (class I, IIa) for which safety and performance can be adequately demonstrated by a combination of nonclinical data (i.e., bench testing and animal testing) and clinical data that already exists on the device (published or unpublished) or by analogy with published data generated on an equivalent device.

Clinical Investigation Route

Specific requirements for clinical evaluation of most devices are not available in the guidance. In the absence of such specific requirements, the manufacturer must decide which data are sufficient for CE marking (number of subjects, type of study design, primary and secondary endpoints, type and schedule of assessments, minimum patient follow-up period, etc.). The Notified Body may be consulted with prior to initiating the clinical trial to verify whether or not the protocol is designed to yield adequate data for CE marking. The objective of a CE marking trial is to demonstrate safety and performance. Therefore the majority of these trials are nonrandomized, single arm, feasibility studies involving less than 100 patients for which the primary objective is to demonstrate safety.

US Approach

The approval process for medical devices in the United States is very different, especially in terms of the scope and size of clinical trials required for high-risk devices. To receive approval to market a device in the European Union, the manufacturer must demonstrate that the device is safe and that it performs in a manner consistent with the manufacturer's intended use. To receive approval to market a class III high-risk (and some class II) device in the United States, the manufacturer must demonstrate that the device is reasonably safe and effective. This typically requires a prospective, randomized controlled, adequately powered clinical trial involving hundreds of patients.

CHALLENGES TO CE MARK STUDIES

Where to Perform the Clinical Study?

- Consider the need for speed, cost, and support in markets.
- For speed, choose a large patient population, and countries with quick regulatory processes.
- For cost, choose less utilized facilities and country.
- For support in markets, in country studies may be helpful.

Difference in Purpose of Study

- In the United States data collected to prove safety and effectiveness (clinical endpoint).
- Outside the United States, data collected to evaluate safety and performance (technical endpoint).

Regulatory Requirements for European Studies

- Comply with GCP
    ICH GCP
    ISO 14155 standards
- Submit for approval by the competent authority.

Good Clinical Practice (GCP)

- Responsibility of investigators to produce and record study data.
- Responsibility of sponsor to monitoring study data.
- Responsibility of ethical committee review to protect human rights and obtain ICF from study participants.

Competent Authority

- Reviews study protocol and informed consent.
- Reviews summary of prior studies (bench, animal, and any human studies).
- Reviews evidence of substantial compliance to Essential Requirements of the medical device directive.
- Responds in 60 days.
- Issues EC approval.

Data Collection

- Capture all data required by the protocol.
- Don't record extraneous data.
- Standardize responses where possible:
    Multiple choice responses
    Ranges
    Norma/abnormal
- Allow space for comments

Requirements of Accepted Devices

- Device is safe.
- Risk of device is acceptable compared with benefit.
- Device performs as intended.

Safety Determination

- By risk analysis.
- By safety throughout the device life span.
- By preventing and managing issues and any problem with safety.

Challenging FDA PMA Cases

This chapter considers a number of challenging FDA PMA cases:

- Use of a subjective endpoint as the primary endpoint. As the subjective endpoint, easing the pain of angina sufferers in class IV heart failure patients was used in PMA P970029 (TMR— transmyocardial revascularization by laser) for two reasons:

  Angina was a characteristic of the patient population and the claim of the study.

  The sponsor provided assurance that maximized determination of this endpoint and also the limit bias.

- Use of historic control as the control group. Historic control was used in the ACCUNET "carotid stent" submission to the FDA for treatment of carotid disease. The PMA was approved by the FDA despite the use of historic control for two reasons:

  Both the sponsor and FDA agreed on OPC for the historic control.

  The historic control was validated by other studies published around the time of submission.

- Utilization of a surrogate endpoint instead of a clinical endpoint: A surrogate endpoint of angiographic late loss was used as the primary endpoint instead of a clinical endpoint in drug-eluting stents.

The Design and Management of Medical Device Clinical Trials: Strategies and Challenges, by Salah Abdel-aleem
Copyright © 2010 John Wiley & Sons, Inc.

PMA P970029 (TMR 2000 HOLMIUM LASER SYSTEM)[56]

This study was undertaken to evaluate the safety and effectiveness of laser treatment for trans myocardial revascularization (TMR) in class IV heart failure patients. It should be noted that patients enrolled in this study were diagnosed as having inoperable coronary artery disease. The patients presented a very diffuse pattern of atherosclerotic disease throughout their coronary circulatory system, and were at the end-stage point of coronary disease. These patients, for the most part, had profound physical limitations due to their angina. So TMR was a new technology for patients with no therapeutic alternatives. In this study angina assessment was based on subjective measurements, and patients were not masked to the treatment. While there was still the possibility that patients exaggerated the intensity of their pain in answering the questions, the sponsor tried to limit this bias by allowing this endpoint to be assessed by independent clinical reviewers from the study who were also masked to the treatment. The panel members were assured about the effectiveness of the TMR in the treatment of those patients but were concerned about the safety of the TMR, particularly because of an early higher rate of mortality in the TMR group (30-day death rate of 5.3% in the TMR versus 1.6% in the medical management group). They were also concerned about the criteria assigned to rollover patients from medical management to the TMR group. The exact mechanism of improving angina pain by TMR was unknown, since there is no clinical correlation between angina and thallium improvement. The following theories were postulated to explain how this therapy might work: (1) it keeps open a channel in the patient, (2) it enhances angiogenesis, (3) it de-enervates the heart, and (4) it has a placebo effect. However, full recognition of the device's mechanism of action was not required for approval of the therapy.

Device Description

The Eclipse TMR Holmium Laser System is composed of the Eclipse TMR 2000 Holmium: YAG laser, fiber-optic delivery systems, and hand pieces. The laser radiation emitted from this system has a wavelength of approximately 2.1 microns, which is in the mid-infrared (invisible) range of electromagnetic spectrum. Water is the target absorber for this laser wavelength. The laser emits 200 microsecond laser radiation pulses at a 5 Hertz pulse repetition rate. The maximum average power is 20 Watts (4 Joules/pulse), while typical clinical levels are in the 6 to 8 Watt range (1.2–1.6 Joules/pulse). These pulses are not synchronized with the cardiac cycles, and there is no visible aiming beam. The laser energy is delivered to the target tissue via fiber optics.

Study Overview   This study was a prospective, multicenter, randomized comparison of laser transmyocardial revascularization as opposed to medical management in class IV angina patients who are not an option for PTCA or CABG intervention. A total of 275 patients were randomized in the study: 132 were randomized to TMR and 143 were randomized to medical management at 18 US sites. The follow-up time points were at 3, 6, and 12 months. The rational for the study was based on the notion that despite 885,000 PTCA or CABG procedures performed annually, there is still 12% of these patients are not considered candidates for interventional procedures due to their vascular system anatomy. So a clear need exists for a new therapy in treating their condition.

Inclusion/Exclusion Criteria   The main inclusion criteria for the study were class IV angina (based on a Canadian Cardiovascular Society classification), namely patients unable to perform any physical activity without chest pain, and with chest pain at rest (the sort of patient who has pain brushing their teeth); these patients were not candidates for re-vascularization, had an EF > 25%, and an area of reversible ischemia. Patients were excluded from the study if they had had a Q-wave MI within the previous three weeks, or a non–Q-wave MI within the previous two weeks; if they were severely unstable (i.e., unweanable from IV anti-anginal medication); If they had uncontrolled ventricular tachy-arrhythmia, or if they had decompensate cardiac failure. Also excluded were patients who had severe COPD; who required chronic anticoagulant medication such as coumadin; who had ventricular mural thrombus, which could, of course, be dislodged during the procedure; and who had a contraindication to dipyridamole, which was used as the stressor in the thallium stress tests.

The Primary Objective   Angina improvement, the primary endpoint in this study, was judged according to the Canadian Cardiovascular Society classification. Improvement was designated as two classes or more improvement. Patients were class IV at baseline, and so they were to have improved to class II or better to be judged as to have improved in the study. An independent core lab at the Cleveland Clinic was used to evaluate the primary endpoint, which was based on two masked interviewers. The secondary endpoints were those of mortality, event-free survival, re-hospitalizations for cardiac causes, myocardial infarction, and medication usage or revascularization attempts such as PTCA or CABG. Two further endpoints were added later in the study, those of exercise treadmill tests and functional status as judged by the Duke Activity Status Index, or DASI questionnaire. For the functional status endpoint, as the Duke Activity Status Index (DASI), questionnaire was used. This is a validated questionnaire and correlates well with oxygen consumption. It consists of 12 questions that are weighted and enable a judgment of the functional status of a patient by summing the weighted score based on these questions.

Treatment failure in this study was defined a priori in consultation with the FDA, scientific advisors of the sponsor, and investigators in the study. It was an objective measure of when patients had failed the treatment to which they were originally randomized. It was defined in this study as the occurrence of one or more of the following events: death, or Q-wave myocardial infarction; two cardiac hospitalizations within three months; three cardiac hospitalizations within a year; or if the patient was unweanable from IV anti-angina after at least 48 hours and two attempts at weaning. Of the 143 patients who were randomized to medical management, 46 patients met the treatment failure criteria and withdrew from this study, that is, became unstable and enrolled in the separate study for unstable patients. Thus at the time of the analysis there were 132 patients who were originally randomized to TMR and who received that therapy; 97 patients who were originally randomized to medical management and who remained on medical management for the duration of the study; and 46 patients who were originally randomized to medical management but who eventually received TMR (Figure 7.1).

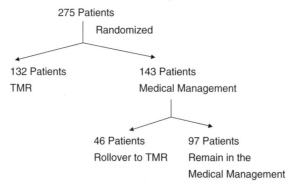

Figure 7.1   TMR study design

Patient Enrollment and Disposition

Safety analysis in this study (e.g. event-free survival, treatment failure, and cardiac re-hospitalizations) was based on intent-to-treat analysis. The 132 TMR patients were compared with the 143 patients originally randomized to medical management. This analysis was used for endpoints that were determined prior to the patient rollover and could therefore not have been impacted by the fact that some of the medical management patients eventually received TMR. To account for patients in the medical management arm who rolled over to TMR, they were censored from the analysis at the time that they rolled over to TMR. Therefore in this analysis the 132 patients originally randomized were compared to medical management with the 97 medical management patients who remained on that therapy for the duration of the study. In these analyses also the 46 rollover patients were included for descriptive purposes only as they were not included in the statistical comparison between the two groups. The rollover censored method of analysis was used for the following endpoints: mortality, angina improvement, perfusion, medication usage, functional status as measured by the DASI survey, and exercise treadmill tests.

Observed Adverse Events

The randomized trial of TMR using the Eclipse TMR System as opposed to Medical Management (MM) involved 275 patients who were followed for a total of 204 patients per year. Among the adverse events reported in this study, as shown in Table 7.1, there was one intra-operative death in the TMR group that occurred in a patient who did not receive TMR—the patient developed ventricular fibrillation that could not be reversed during preparation for TMR. Within 30 days of TMR, five other patients died of cardiac causes and one died of pulmonary causes. In the MM group, two patients died within 30 days of enrollment in the study, both due to cardiac causes. During 12 month follow-up, an additional 9 patients in the TMR arm died (6 due to cardiac causes, one each due to renal causes, multisystem organ failure, and sudden death), and an additional 5 patients died in the MM arm (all due to cardiac causes). Adverse events were reviewed by an independent, masked **Data** Safety and Monitoring Board (DSMB).

The following events were reported only once in patients treated with TMR: allergic reaction, grand mal seizure, hemothorax, cardiomyopathy, pericarditis, peripheral edema, pneumothorax, and pulmonary

TABLE 7.1 Adverse Events Reported in the TMR Study

	TMR (N = 132)		MM (N = 143)	
	Early	Total	Early	Total
Adverse event	(0–30 days)	(0 days to 1 yr)	(0–30 days)	(0 days to 1 yr)
Any adverse event	39% (51)	55% (72)	22% (31)	56% (80)
Angina/chest pain Requiring re-hospitalization	2.3% (3)	17% (22)	16% (23)	44% (63)
Arrhythmia, atrial	9.8% (13)	11% (14)	0.7% (1)	0.7% (1)
Arrhythmia, operative ventricular fibrillation (OP VF)	8.3% (11)	NA	NA	NA
Arrhythmia, other ventricular arrhythmia	12% (16)	13% (17)	0% (0)	0% (0)
Congestive heart failure	3.8% (5)	5.3% (7)	1.4% (2)	4.2% (6)
Death (all causes)	5.3% (7)	13%[a]	1.6% (2)	8.6%[a]
Dyspnea	0% (0)	0% (0)	1.4% (2)	8.4% (12)
Hypotension	9.8% (13)	11% (14)	0% (0)	0% (0)
Q-wave MI	0.8% (1)	1.7%[a]	0.8% (1)	3.8%[a]
Non–Q-wave MI	4.5% (6)	12%[a]	0.8% (1)	6.7%[a]
Pleural effusion	0% (0)	2.3% (3)	0% (0)	0% (0)
Respiratory insufficiency	3.0% (4)	3.0% (4)	0% (0)	0% (0)
Systemic infection	1.5% (2)	1.5% (2)	0% (0)	0% (0)
Transfusion required for other reasons than TMR	1.5%[b] (2)	1.5% (2)	0% (0)	0% (0)
Unstable requiring I.V. Anti-anginals	1.5% (2)	17% (22)	19% (27)	48% (68)

Note: All patients in the randomized trial (N = 275).
[a]Survival estimated using Kaplan–Meier methods.
[b]1 due to GI bleed, 1 due to preexisting anemia.

embolus. The following events were reported only once in patients treated with MM: cardiogenic shock, dehydration, and pneumonia. As shown in Table 7.1, atrial and ventricular arrhythmia, hypotension, and death within 30 days were higher in TMR as compared to the MM arm. In contrast, the percentage of unstable patients requiring I.V. anti-anginal agents was higher in the MM arm than the TMR group.

Potential Adverse Events

Adverse events potentially associated with the use of TMR include:

- Accidental laser hit
- Congestive heart failure
- Acute myocardial infarction
- Death
- Arrhythmia
- Mitral valve damage
- Cerebrovascular accident
- Pulmonary complications
- Conduction pathway injury
- Unstable angina

Patient baseline characteristics and cardiac risk factors such as diabetes, smoking, hypertension, hypercholesterolemia, and a history of MI are shown in Table 7.2.

As shown in Table 7.2 the baseline demographics and clinical history characteristics between the TMR and MM groups were comparable. Table 7.3 lists the principal safety and effectiveness results. There was statistically significant difference in angina improvement, and 12-month survival (event-free, freedom from treatment failure, and freedom from cardiac re-hospitalization). There were no apparent differences in perfusion as measured by thallium scans. The Kaplan–Meier survival estimates at 12 months were similar between the two groups: 87% for TMR treated patients and 91% for MM patients.

Angina Improvement   Angina improvement was defined as improvement in angina symptoms from baseline by at least two angina classes, as judged by the Canadian Cardiovascular Society's definition of angina. All patients had class IV angina at baseline. The results of angina class improvement as function of follow-up time are shown in Table 7.4. There were significants increases in the number of patients with improved angina class in the TMR arm as compared to MM arm at 3, 6, and 12 months of follow-up.

Quality of Life   Quality of life was assessed at 12 months using the Duke Activity Status Index (DASI) questionnaire. The DASI questionnaire consists of 12 questions about activities that represent major aspects of physical function, including personal care, ambulation,

TABLE 7.2 Patient Baseline Characteristics and Cardiac Risk Factors

	TMR	MM	Difference (TMR – MM) [CI]
N = patients	132	143	
Male	74% (98)	76% (108)	–2% [–12%, 9%]
Age (years)	60 ± 10	60 ± 11	0 [–0.2, 0.2]
Mean ± SD	(32,83)	(35,82)	
Range {min, max}			
Ejection fraction (%)	47 ± 10	47 ± 10	0 1 [–0.2, 0.2]
Mean ± SD			
Range {min, max}	{25, 77}	{25, 70}	
History of diabetes	46% (60/131)	48% (68)	–2% [–14%, 10%]
History of smoking	72% (95)	72% (101/141)	0% [–10%, 11%]
History of hypertension	70% (92)	71% (98/138)	–1% [–12%, 10%]
History of hypercholesterolemia	79% (100/126)	84% (110/131)	–5% [–14%, 5%]
Family history of CAD before age 55			
Yes	50% (66)	45% (64)	5% [–7%, 17%]
No	29% (38)	22% (32)	7% [–4%, 17%]
Unknown	21% (28)	33% (47)	–12% [–22%, –1%]
History of MI	64% (85)	64% (91/142)	0% [–11%, 12%]
Documented Q-wave MI	16% (21)	16% (23/142)	0% [–9%, 8%]
History of CHF	17% (22/129)	26% (34/132)	–9% [–19%, 1%]
Previous PTCA	48% (63)	48% (68)	0% [–12%, 12%]
Previous CABG	86% (113)	86% (123)	0% [–9%, 8%]
History of either PTCA intervention or CABG	92% (121)	87% (125)	5% [–3%, 12%]

Note: Unless otherwise specified, the denominator was the total n for each specified group. There were no statistically significant difference (p > 0.05) between these groups. p-Value calculated using Fisher's exact test. Two-sided, chi-square and Student's *t*-test. CI = 95% confidence Interval by normal approximation.

household tasks, sexual function, and recreational activities. Each answer has a weight associated with it, and the patients' weighted answers were summed to generate the DASI score. The highest possible score is 58.2. At 12 months, TMR patients had a mean DASI score of 21, which was statistically significantly better than the MM patients whose mean score was 12 ($p = 0.003$).

Exercise Treadmill Testing At 12 months follow-up, TMR patients were able to perform a statistically significantly greater workload (as measured in METS) than MM patients. TMR patients were able to perform an average of 5.0 METS, compared with 3.9 METS for MM patients. TMR patients were able to exercise an average of 7.9 minutes

TABLE 7.3 Safety and Effectiveness Results

	TMR (N = 132)	MM (N = 143)	Difference (TMR − MM) [CI]
Angina improvement at 12 months	76% (58/76)	32% (16/50)	44%* [28%, 60%]
Thallium scan results at 12 months (N = 61)			
Mean ± SD Δ extent ischemia (%)	−0.9 ± 9.4	−0.6 ± 10.8	−0.3 [−5.0, 5.6]
Mean ± SD Δ extent rest defects (%)	1.6 ± 12.5	2.2 ± 11.8	−0.6 [−5.9, 7.1]
Freedom from all cause mortality			
30-day survival	95%	98%	3.7% [−1%, 8%]
Survival at 12 months (KM)	87%	91%	4.9% [−2.5%, 12.3%]
Event free survival at 12 months (KM)	55%	31%	24%* [12%. 35%]
Freedom from treatment failure at 12 months (KM)	74%	48%	26%* [16%, 38%]
Freedom from hospitalization for cardiac Causes at 12 months (KM)	61%	33%	28%* [17%, 39%]
Medication use at 12 months			
Decrease in calcium channel blockers (% Pts)	56%	24%	32%* [14%, 50%]
Decrease in beta blockers (% Pts)	39%	17%	22%* [6%, 39%]
Decrease in nitrates (% pts)	39%	24%	15% [−2%, 31%]
Quality of life (DASI score) at 12 months	21 ± 14	12 ± 11	9* [3.1, 14.9]
Exercise treadmill tests at 12 months			
Total exercise time (minutes)	7.9 ± 4.5	6.2 ± 5.6	1.71 [−0.6, 4.0]
Total workload (METS)	5.0 ± 0.7	3.9 ± 0.8	1.1* [0.0, 2.1]

Note:
- * = <0.05 p-value calculated using Fisher's exact test, two-sided for proportions, Students t-test, two-sided for continuous variables, or log rank test for KM survival estimates.
- KM: Kaplan–Meier survival estimates.
- CI 95% confidence interval by normal approximation.
- Angina improvement: Improvement In angina symptoms from baseline to 12 months by 2 Canadian Society classes whose patients were available at 12-month follow-up.
- Thallium scans: A negative value indicates an Improvement In a parameter; a positive value Indicates a worsening.
- Event-free survival: Freedom from death, Q-wave Ml, hosptilization for cardiac causes, coronary artery bypass graft (CABG), or percutaneous intervention.
- Treatment failure: Death, Q-wave Ml, 2 cardiac hosptilizations within 3 months, 3 cardiac hosptilizations within 1 year, or unweanable from IV anti-anginal mediations for at least 48 hours after at least 2 attempts at weaning.
- DASI: Duke Activity Status Index for quality of life. A higher score indicates a better quality of life.

TABLE 7.4 Improvements in the Angina Class

Angina Improvement	TMR	MM	Difference (TMR − MM) [CI]	p-Value (TMR vs. MM)
3 Months	33% (95/115)	13% (13/95)	70% [60%, 79%]	<0.0001
6 Months	86% (84/98)	20% (15/74)	66% [54%,77%]	<0.0001
12 Months	76% (58/76)	32% (16/50)	44% [28%, 60%]	<0.0001

Note: *p*-Value is calculated using Fisher's exact test, two-sided. CI = 95% confidence interval by normal approximation.

compared with 6.2 minutes for MM patients, but this difference was statistically nonsignificant.

Morbidity and Mortality There was one intra-operative death in the TMR group, which occurred in a patient who did not receive TMR. Within 30 days of TMR, 5 other patients died of cardiac causes and one died of pulmonary causes. In the MM group, 2 patients died within 30 days of enrollment in the study, both due to cardiac causes. During 12 month follow-up, an additional 9 patients in the TMR arm died (6 due to cardiac causes, 1 each due to renal causes, multisystem organ failure, and sudden death), and an additional 5 patients died in the MM arm (all due to cardiac causes). Kaplan–Meier survival estimates at 12 months were similar for the two groups: 87% for TMR treated patients and 91% for MM patients. In the TMR group, 5 of 23 patients treated prior to July, 1996 died within 30 days of the procedure. Investigators attributed this result to "fluid loading" patients prior to the TMR procedure. This practice of "fluid loading" was discontinued in June 1996. From July 1996 to completion of enrollment in July 1998, an additional 109 patients received TMR in the study. In this group 30 day mortality was 1.8% (2/109).

Treatment Failure Treatment failure was defined in this study as the occurrence of at least one of the following events: death, Q-wave MI, 2 cardiac hospitalizations within 3 months, 3 cardiac hospitalizations within 1 year, or unweanable from IV anti-anginal medications for at least 48 hours after at least 2 attempts at weaning. According to the Kaplan–Meier survival estimates, a significantly higher percentage of TMR patients (74%) had not experienced treatment failure at 12 months, compared with MM patients (48%) ($p < 0.0001$).

MM Patients Rolled over to TMR Of the 143 patients randomized to MM, 46 patients met treatment failure criteria, became unstable, and withdrew from the randomized study. These 46 patients then enrolled in a separate study for unstable patients and received TMR. These patients were referred to as rollover patients. The mean time to rollover was 81 days. Peri-operative mortality (within 30 days of the TMR procedure) occurred in 4 (8.7%) rollover patients. There were no additional deaths during the 12-month follow-up period in the rollover group. At the 12-month follow-up, 78% (29/37) of the rollover patients experienced angina improvement.

Conclusions Drawn from the Study   Data from the multicenter clinical trial show treatment with the Eclipse TMR Holmium Laser System provides a reduction in the severity of angina in the majority of patients, but the risks of the procedure (including major cardiac arrhythmias and early death within 30 days of the operation) were higher. After one year had elapsed, the overall mortality was similar between the treated and control groups. Experience beyond one year is not yet available.

Panel Recommendation

At the advisory meeting held on October27, 1998, the Circulatory System Devices Panel recommended that the Eclipse TMR Holmium Laser System be submitted for approval to the Center for Devices and Radiological Health (CDRH) of the following:

1. Changes to Indications for usage, warnings and precautions, and patient counseling information sections of the Information for Use (labeling).
2. Postapproval study to further define the 30-day postoperative mortality predictors (risk factors), effectiveness as a function of operator experience (the learning curve), and the medical conditions treated.

The postapproval study was to enroll 600 consecutive patients at all centers to assess clinical status, including mortality. A detailed protocol and statistical analysis plan was to be submitted to the agency in the form of a PMA supplement for review and approval within 30 days of the date of the approval order. Prior to initiation of the postapproval study, treatment of patients was to be limited to 90 days after the date of the submission letter and to total 90 patients. Once the postapproval study was initiated, the restrictions on the number of patients would be removed.

TABLE 7.5 Overview of the ARCHeR Trials

	ARCHeR 1	ARCHeR 2	ARCHeR 3
Products evaluated	Over-the-wire ACCULINK™ Carotid Stent System	Over-the-wire ACCULINK™ and over-the-wire ACCUNET™ systems	Rapid exchange ACCULINK™ and rapid exchange ACCUNET™ systems
Study design	Nonrandomized, multicenter, single-arm, prospective clinical trials		
Sample size	158 (plus 51 lead-in patients)[5]	278 (plus 25 lead-in patients)[5]	145 Patients
Number of sites	25 Sites in the United States	37 Sites in the United States and 1 site in South America	19 Sites in the United States, 4 sites in Europe, and 1 site in South America
Primary endpoint	30-Day death, stroke, MI and ipsilateral stroke at 31–365 days	30-Day death, stroke, and MI and ipsilateral stroke at 31–365 days; ACCUNET™ device success[2]	30-Day death, stroke, and MI
Secondary endpoints— all trials	Device success[1,2]—clinical success[3]—target lesion revascularization—access site complications requiring treatment		
Specific secondary endpoints	Six and 12-month ultrasound (annually thereafter)	Six and 12-month ultrasound (annually thereafter)—medical resource utilization	Six and 12-month ultrasound— ipsilateral stroke between 31 and 365 days[4]
Study hypothesis	Noninferiority to historical control	Noninferiority to historical control	Noninferiority to ARCHeR 2 results at 30 days
Patient follow-up	Neurologic evaluation by an independent neurologist and patient assessment at 24 hours, 30 days, 6 months, 12 months (every 6 months thereafter for ARCHeR 1 and 2 only)—TIA / Stroke Questionnaire and adverse event assessment at 30 days and 3, 6, 9, and 12 months. ECG at 30 days, ultrasound at 30 days, 6 and 12 months (annually thereafter for ARCHeR 1 and 2 only)		

[1]Attainment of final result, <50% residual stenosis covering an area no longer than the original lesion, using the ACCULINK™ System as described in the protocol.

[2]Device delivered, placed, and retrieved as described in the protocol.

[3]ACCULINK™ device/procedure success without death, emergency endarterectomy, repeat PTA/ thrombolysis of the target vessel, stroke, or MI within seven days of the procedure.

[4]Data collection for the ARCHeR 3 study is not complete beyond 30 days. Secondary endpoints have not been evaluated.

[5]ARCHeR 1 and 2 trials each had a lead-in phase for initial clinical experience. An additional 76 patients were enrolled in this phase of the clinical study, 51 in ARCHeR 1 and 25 in ARCHeR 2. The natures and frequencies of endpoints and adverse events reported in lead-in patients were consistent with those reported in the pivotal trials, and thus are not reported here.

PMA P040012 CAROTID STENTING FOR TREATING CAROTID ARTERY DISEASE

Acculink™ and RX ACCULINK™ Carotid Stent System[57]

Study Design   The ACCULINK for Revascularization of Carotids in High-Risk Patients (ARCHeR) Clinical Trials were a series of prospective, nonrandomized, multicenter, single-arm clinical trials. These trials were performed to demonstrate the safety and efficacy of the ACCULINK™ and RX ACCULINK™ Carotid Stent Systems with embolic protection to treat high-risk surgical and nonsurgical symptomatic (≥50% stenosis) and asymptomatic (≥80% stenosis) subjects with disease in the internal carotid artery. A total of 581 patients were enrolled at 45 clinical sites in the United States and five sites outside the United States in these registries. An overview of the design of this trial is presented in Table 7.5. The design of the trial was as follows:

ARCHeR 1   Evaluated the over-the-wire (OTW) ACCULINK™ Carotid Stent System and included 158 registry patients. The primary objective of the study was to determine if the occurrence rate of the composite primary endpoint of stroke, death, and myocardial infarction (MI) at 30 days and ipsilateral stroke at one year for carotid stenting is not inferior to the occurrence rate of carotid endarterectomy (CEA) in the population under evaluation.

ARCHeR 2   Evaluated the OTW ACCULINK™ Carotid Stent System and OTW ACCUNET™ Embolic Protection System and included 278 registry patients. The primary objective of the study was the same as in ARCHeR 1. A second primary endpoint for this study was ACCUNET™ device success.

ARCHeR 3   Evaluated the rapid exchange (RX) ACCULINK™ Carotid Stent System and RX ACCUNET™ Embolic Protection System and included 145 patients. The primary objective of the study was to establish equivalence (noninferiority) to the ARCHeR 2 results with respect to 30-day death, stroke, and MI as a means of establishing equivalency between the OTW and RX devices.

HISTORIC CONTROL ASSUMPTIONS

The historic control for this trial was based on OPC that was derived from multiple clinical studies, including the following land mark studies:

- NASCET[58], North American Symptomatic Carotid Endarterectomy Trial. Methods, patient characteristics, and progress.
- North American Symptomatic Carotid Endarterectomy Trial[59].
- ACAS[60], Endarterectomy for asymptomatic carotid artery stenosis. Executive Committee for the Asymptomatic Carotid Atherosclerosis Study.

The OPC proposed for these studies continued to be validated by newly published studies, particularly the SAPPHIRE trial[61] which was presented to the FDA few months before the ACCULINK PMA submission.

The study hypothesis of the ARCHeR 1 and ARCHeR 2 trials was to show equivalence (noninferiority) between carotid stenting and a historic control, based on the standard of care. The historic control was established based on a review of the current literature on carotid endarterectomy and medical therapy. From this review the rate of 30-day death, stroke, MI and ipsilateral stroke at 31 to 365 days was estimated at 15% for patients with medical comorbidities, and estimated at 11% for patients with anatomy unfavorable for carotid endarterectomy (CEA). A weighted historic control (WHC) was calculated based on the proportion of each of these patient groups enrolled in the study.

$$WHC = pc * 15\% + pa * 11\%$$

where pc = the proportion of patients with medical co-morbidities, and pa = the proportion of patients with unfavorable anatomy. Using this equation, the WHC rate at one year was calculated for both ARCHeR 1 and ARCHeR 2 to be 14.5%. The ARCHeR 3 trial was designed to demonstrate equivalence (noninferiority) of the safety and performance of the rapid exchange RX ACCULINK™ and RX ACCUNET™ systems to results observed in the ARCHeR 2 trial for the OTW ACCULINK™ and ACCUNET™ systems based on 30-day results.

The primary objectives of the ARCHeR 1 and ARCHeR 2 trials were met. The upper confidence limits for primary endpoint rates fell below the 14.5% WHC for both studies, demonstrating that carotid stenting is noninferior to carotid endarterectomy in the studied high-risk population.

The primary objective of the ARCHeR 3 study, that the 30-day primary endpoint for the ARCHeR 3 study was noninferior to that of the ARCHeR 2 study, was met. The upper bound of the 95% confidence interval of the difference between ARCHeR 3 and ARCHeR 2 is 4.75%, which is less than the delta of 8% ($p = 0.005$). Thus results from ARCHeR 3 are determined to be noninferior to those of ARCHeR 2, and the RX and OTW devices are determined to yield similar clinical results.

The ACCULINK™ Carotid Stent System and the RX ACCULINK™ Carotid Stent System, used in conjunction with Guidant carotid embolic protection systems, is indicated for the treatment of patients at high risk for adverse events from carotid endarterectomy who require carotid revascularization and meet the criteria outlined below:

1. Patients with neurological symptoms and ≥50% stenosis of the common or internal carotid artery by ultrasound or angiogram *or* patients without neurological symptoms and ≥80% stenosis of the common or internal carotid artery by ultrasound or angiogram, *and*
2. Patients must have a reference vessel diameter within the range of 4.0 and 9.0 mm at the target lesion. The key point of this PMA was that the submission of the PMA was based in three nonrandomized registries and the control group was selected as a historic control.

An overview of the ARCHeR trials is presented in Table 7.5.

Serious adverse events that occurred in the ARCHeR trials at ≤30 days, and from 31 to 365 days, are presented in Tables 7.6, and 7.7,

TABLE 7.6 Serious Adverse Events Summary at ≤30 Days

Event categories[1,2]	ARCHeR 2 (N = 278)		ARCHeR 3 (N = 145)		p-Value[3]	ARCHeR 1 (N = 158)	
	n	%	n	%		n	%
All death, stroke, and MI[4]	23	8.27	11	7.59	0.824	12	7.59
Death	6	2.16	2	1.38	0.625	4	2.53
Stroke-related	2	0.72	0	0.00	0.406	1	0.63
Not stroke-related	4	1.44	2	1.38	0.965	3	1.90
Ipsilateral stroke	14	5.04	7	4.83	0.933	6	3.80
Major	3	1.08	2	1.38	0.802	2	1.27
Minor[4]	11	3.96	5	3.45	0.816	4	2.53
Non-ipsilateral stroke	1	0.36	1	0.69	0.653	1	0.63
Non-stroke neurological	6	2.16	1	0.69	0.341	3	1.90
Target lesion revascularization (TLR), clinically indicated	0	0.00	0	0.00	1.000	0	0.00
Cardiac	23	8.27	13	8.97	0.826	22	13.92
MI	8	2.88	2	1.38	0.406	4	2.53
Arrhythmia	3	1.08	3	2.07	0.433	4	2.53
Angina	3	1.08	3	2.07	0.433	1	0.63
Congestive heart failure (CHF)	5	1.80	4	2.76	0.542	4	2.53
Coronary artery disease (CAD)	0	0.00	1	0.69	0.087	3	1.90

TABLE 7.6 *Continued*

Event categories[1,2]	ARCHeR 2 (N = 278)		ARCHeR 3 (N = 145)		p-Value[3]	ARCHeR 1 (N = 158)	
	n	%	n	%		n	%
Procedural complication	27	9.71	8	5.52	0.194	11	6.96
Hypotension	15	5.40	2	1.38	0.092	6	3.80
Arrhythmia	11	3.96	0	0.00	0.048	5	3.16
Vasospasm	4	1.44	0	0.00	0.238	0	0.00
Dissection[5]	2	0.72	3	2.07	0.223	0	0.00
In-stent thrombosis	1	0.36	1	0.69	0.653	0	0.00
Emergent CEA[6]	2	0.72	0	0.00	0.406	0	0.00
Emergent intervention[7]	1	0.36	1	0.69	0.653	0	0.00
Access site complication	13	4.68	4	2.76	0.405	9	5.70
Requiring repair/transfusion	8	2.88	2	1.38	0.406	6	3.80
Vascular	3	1.08	0	0.00	0.308	2	1.27
Hemodynamic	6	2.16	4	2.76	0.722	3	1.90
Bleeding	7	2.52	6	4.14	0.387	11	6.96
Requiring transfusion	5	1.80	5	3.45	0.310	9	5.70
GI bleeding	0	0.00	2	1.38	0.015	2	1.27
Blood dyscrasia	5	1.80	2	1.38	0.776	0	0.00
Respiratory	5	1.80	0	0.00	0.186	2	1.27
Gastrointestinal	2	0.72	0	0.00	0.406	0	0.00
Genitourinary	1	0.36	1	0.69	0.653	1	0.63
Infection	4	1.44	0	0.00	0.238	1	0.63
Metabolic	5	1.80	0	0.00	0.186	1	0.63
Musculoskeletal	0	0.00	0	0.00	1.000	1	0.63
Miscellaneous[8]	0	0.00	0	0.00	1.000	3	1.90

[1]Patients who had multiple events could be counted in more than one category/subcategory of an event. Counts represent the number of patients who experienced one or more events.

[2]Three of the reported adverse events were related to device failures/malfunctions. The three are described below in notes 5 through 7.

[3]Because of the multiple tests of significance performed, the individual test level for significance was set conservatively at $p < 0.01$ after a Bonferroni adjustment. Therefore none of the AE rates were deemed significantly different statistically between ARCHeR 2 and ARCHeR 3.

[4]Two patients suffered strokes that were determined to be nonserious adverse events. However, because the events did not meet the criteria for a serious adverse event (no intervention to prevent permanent impairment, no persistent or significant disability), they are not included in this table. The events are included as strokes in the composite endpoints.

[5]One dissection in the ARCHeR 2 study was attributed by the physician to the OTW ACCUNET™ System. The physician was not able to cross the lesion with the device.

[6]One CEA in the ARCHeR 2 study resulted when the OTW ACCUNET™ System became entangled with the deployed stent and could not be retrieved by the physician.

[7]The emergent intervention in the ARCHeR 3 study resulted when the RX ACCUNET™ filter basket became entangled with the deployed stent and detached from the guide wire during the retrieval attempt. The physician opted to stent the basket in place in the artery. No additional adverse events related to this device malfunction were reported as of the last patient follow-up (9 months postprocedure).

[8]The three miscellaneous adverse events reported in the ARCHeR 1 study were bladder tumor, headache, and rash.

TABLE 7.7   Serious Adverse Events Summary, up to 365 Days[1]

Event Categories[2,3]	31–365 Days				0–365 Days			
	ARCHeR 1 (N = 154)		ARCHeR 2 (N = 272)		ARCHeR 1 (N = 158)		ARCHeR 2 (N = 278)	
	n	%	n	%	n	%	n	%
Death	10	6.49	18	6.62	14	8.86	24	8.63
Stroke-related	0	0.00	1	0.37	1	0.63	3	1.08
Not stroke-related	8	5.19	16	5.88	11	6.96	20	7.19
Unknown	2	1.30	1	0.37	2	1.27	1	0.36
Ipsilateral stroke	1	0.65	3	1.10	7	4.43	17	6.12
Major	0	0.00	0	0.00	2	1.27	3	1.08
Minor	1	0.65	3	1.10	5	3.16	14	5.04
Not ipsilateral stroke	1	0.65	3	1.10	2	1.27	4	1.44
Not neurological stroke	1	0.65	3	1.10	4	2.53	9	3.24
Target lesion revascularization (TLR), clinically indicated	7	4.55	6	2.21	7	4.43	6	2.16
Cardiac	26	16.88	50	18.38	46	29.11	69	24.82
MI	1	0.65	8	2.94	4	2.53	16	5.76
Arrhythmia	6	3.90	4	1.47	10	6.33	7	2.52
Angina	6	3.90	13	4.78	7	4.43	16	5.76
Congestive heart failure (CHF)	5	3.25	7	2.57	8	5.06	11	3.96
Coronary artery disease (CAD)	6	3.90	6	2.21	9	5.70	6	2.16
Procedural complication	0	0.00	0	0.00	11	6.96	27	9.71
Hypotension	0	0.00	0	0.00	6	3.80	15	5.40
Arrhythmia	0	0.00	0	0.00	5	3.16	11	3.96
Vasospasm	0	0.00	0	0.00	0	0.00	4	1.44
Dissection	0	0.00	0	0.00	0	0.00	1	0.72
In-stent thrombosis	0	0.00	0	0.00	0	0.00	1	0.36
Emergent CEA	0	0.00	0	0.00	0	0.00	2	0.72
Emergent intervention	0	0.00	0	0.00	0	0.00	1	0.36
Access site complication	0	0.00	1	0.37	9	5.70	14	5.04
Requiring repair / transfusion	0	0.00	0	0.00	6	3.80	8	2.88
Vascular	14	9.09	25	9.19	15	9.49	27	9.71
Hemodynamic	4	2.60	4	1.47	7	4.43	10	3.60
Bleeding	0	0.00	3	1.10	11	6.96	10	3.60
Requiring transfusion	0	0.00	2	0.74	9	5.70	7	2.52
GI bleeding	0	0.00	0	0.00	2	1.27	0	0.00
Blood dyscrasia	2	1.30	1	0.37	2	1.27	6	2.16
Respiratory	5	3.25	5	1.84	7	4.43	10	3.60
Gastrointestinal	10	6.49	5	1.84	10	6.33	6	2.16
Genitourinary	0	0.00	1	0.37	1	0.63	2	0.72
Infection	2	1.30	4	1.47	4	2.53	8	2.88

TABLE 7.7 *Continued*

Event Categories[2,3]	31–365 Days				0–365 Days			
	ARCHeR 1 (N = 154)		ARCHeR 2 (N = 272)		ARCHeR 1 (N = 158)		ARCHeR 2 (N = 278)	
	n	%	n	%	n	%	n	%
Metabolic	2	1.30	3	1.10	3	1.90	8	2.88
Musculoskeletal	1	0.65	5	1.84	2	1.27	5	1.80
Miscellaneous[4]	5	3.25	9	3.31	8	5.06	9	3.24

[1]Data >30 days for ARCHeR 3 are not available because not all subjects completed one-year follow-up.
[2]Patients who had multiple events could be counted in more than one category/subcategory of an event. Counts represent the number of patients who have experienced one or more events.
[3]None of the adverse events reported in the period 31 to 365 days were related to device failures/malfunctions.
[4]The 5 miscellaneous adverse events reported in the ARCHeR 1 during the 31 to 365-day period study include hospitalization for planned surgery (1), bladder cancer (1), biopsy (1), nonresponsive episode adjudicated as chronic subdural hematoma (1), and a fall (1). The additional 3 events in the 0- to 365-day period were bladder tumor (1), headache (1), and rash (1). The 9 miscellaneous adverse events reported in the ARCHeR 2 study during the 31- to 365-day period included cancer (4), weakness accompanying a GI bleed (1), glaucoma (1), cataract surgery (1), post-thoracotomy syndrome (1), and hospitalization for elective surgery (1).

TABLE 7.8 **Cause of Death**[1]

Events	ARCHeR 1		ARCHeR 2		ARCHeR 3	
	n	%	n	%	n	%
0–30 Days[2]	*N* = 158		*N* = 278		*N* = 145	
Stroke	1	0.63	2	0.72	0	0.00
Cardiac	3	1.90	4	1.44	1	0.69
Bleeding (GI)	0	0.00	0	0.00	1	0.69
31–365 Days[3]	*N* = 154		*N* = 272		**N/A**[4]	
Stroke	0	0.00	1	0.36		
Cardiac	3	1.94	9	3.31		
Cancer	1	0.65	2	0.74		
Bleeding (GI)	0	0.00	0	0.00		
Respiratory	2	1.30	2	0.74		
Gastrointestinal	0	0.00	1	0.36		
Genitourinary	1	0.65	0	0.00		
Infection	1	0.65	2	0.74		
Unknown	2	1.30	1	0.38		
Total death	**14**	**8.90**	**24**	**8.63**		

[1]None of the reported deaths were due to a device malfunction or failure.
[2]Of the deaths 0 to 30 days, 5 were considered device or procedure related: 3 strokes, 2 cardiac.
[3]Of the deaths 31 to 365 days, 1 was considered device or procedure related: 1 stroke.
[4]Data >30 days for ARCHeR 3 are not available because not all subjects completed one-year follow-up.

TABLE 7.9 Patient Follow-Up

	ARCHeR 1	ARCHeR 2	ARCHeR 3
30 Days			
Patients enrolled	158	278	145
Cumulative death	4	4	2
Cumulative withdrawn or LTF	2	1	1
Patients evaluable	152	273	142
Patients evaluated[1]	152	272	141
Neurological evaluation	128	256	130
Ultrasound evaluation	133	256	136
Other clinical evaluation only[2]	14	10	5
365 Days			
Cumulative death	12	21	
Cumulative withdrawn/LTF	14	11	
Patients evaluable	132	246	
Patients evaluated[1]	131	239	
Neurological evaluation	116	207	
Ultrasound evaluation	121	213	
Other clinical evaluation only[2]	9	19	

[1]Patients who had one or more of the evaluations listed: neurological, ultrasound, or clinical.
[2]Other clinical evaluation includes: office visit, telephone conversation with site, TIA / Stroke Questionnaire, hospitalization.

respectively. Table 7.8 presents the causes of death that occurred in ARCHeR 1, 2, and 3 at 30 days and from 31 to 365 days. The clinical and angiographic patient follow-up for up to 365 days is presented in Table 7.9.

Table 7.10 shows the patient baseline demographic characteristics including baseline lesion and vessel characteristics, high risk medical, surgical, and unfavorable anatomic characteristics.

Tables 7.11 and 7.12 show the assessments of the primary and secondary safety and efficacy endpoints in ARCHeR 1, 2, and 3.

Table 7.12 presents the efficacy assessment event rates for the primary endpoint, such as show the device's technical and clinical success.

CDRH Decision

The FDA issued an approval order in 2004. The RX and OTW ACCULINK Carotid Stent Systems were granted expedited review status because these devices could offer a viable alternative to the current standard of care for patients with carotid artery disease. Because

TABLE 7.10 Baseline Patient Demographics

Demographics and Medical History	ARCHeR 2 (N = 278)	ARCHeR 3 (N = 145)	P value[1]	ARCHeR 1 (N = 158)
Age				
Mean ± SD	70.48 ± 9.38 (278)	71.13 ± 9.40 (145)	0.499	69.21 ± 9.65 (158)
Range (min, max)	(45.29, 92.67)	(38.94, 88.78)		(40.28, 90.14)
Age ≥80 year **gender** male	15.5% (43/278)	17.9% (26/145)	0.579	13.3% (21/158)
Medical history	68.3% (190/278)	68.3% (99/145)	1.000	63.9% (101/158)
Diabetes	39.9% (111/278)	34.5% (50/145)	0.293	37.3% (59/158)
Hypertension	84.2% (234/278)	83.3% (120/144)	0.889	83.5% (132/158)
Hypercholesterolemia	71.9% (200/278)	82.4% (117/142)	0.022	64.7% (101/156)
Current smoker	17.7% (49/277)	17.7% (25/141)	1.000	23.7% (37/156)
Number of symptomatic patients (TIA, stroke or amaurosis fugax within 180 days)	24.1% (67/278)	21.4% (31/145)	0.547	25.3% (40/158)
Baseline Lesion and Vessel Characteristics				
No calcification	50.4% (139/276)	42.3% (60/142)	0.122	64.9% (98/151)
Unilateral calcification	27.2% (75/276)	23.2% (33/142)	0.411	27.2% (41/151)
Bilateral calcification, **lesion length (mm)**	22.5% (62/276)	34.5% (49/142)	0.010	7.9% (12/151)
Mean ± SD (N)	14.55 ± 7.14 (276)	14.84 ± 7.82 (142)	0.707	16.17 ± 7.45 (157)
Range (min, max), **minimum lumen diameter (MLD, mm)**	(0.00, 56.51)	(3.57, 43.81)		(4.72, 50.37)
Mean ± SD (N)	1.35 ± 0.56 (276)	1.21 ± 0.53 (142)	0.013	1.37 ± 0.64 (156)
Range (min, max), **percent diameter stenosis (%DS)**	(0.10, 3.57)	(0.00, 3.03)		(0.10, 3.15)
Mean ± SD (N)	69.93 ± 10.86 (276)	73.04 ± 10.13 (142)	0.005	72.62 ± 10.99 (156)
Range (min, max)	(31.03, 95.95)	(47.40, 100.0)		(42.96, 98.14)
High-risk Inclusion Criteria	*% (n/N)*	*% (n/N)*		*% (n/N)*
Medical/surgical comorbidities				
Two or more diseased coronary arteries	27.7% (77/278)	25.5% (37/145)	0.647	28.5% (45/158)
Unstable angina	7.9% (22/278)	6.9% (10/145)	0.847	7.6% (12/158)
MI prior 30d and need carotid artery revascularization	3.6% (10/278)	2.1% (3/145)	0.556	4.4% (7/158)
Need CABG or valve surgery	14.0% (39/278)	15.2% (22/145)	0.772	19.0% (30/158)
Contralateral occlusion of ICA	16.2% (45/278)	12.4% (18/145)	0.318	20.9% (33/158)

TABLE 7.10 *Continued*

Demographics and Medical History	ARCHeR 2 (N = 278)	ARCHeR 3 (N = 145)	P value[1]	ARCHeR 1 (N = 158)
On list for major organ transplant	0.0% (0/278)	0.7% (1/145)	0.343	0.0% (0/158)
Ejection fraction <30% or NYHA = III	38.8% (108/278)	27.6% (40/145)	0.024	29.7% (47/158)
$FEV_1 < 30\%$ (predicted)	3.2% (9/278)	4.8% (7/145)	0.429	5.1% (8/158)
Dialysis-dependent renal failure	2.2% (6/278)	2.1% (3/145)	1.000	5.1% (8/158)
Uncontrolled diabetes	0.0% (0/278)	0.7% (1/145)	0.343	0.0% (0/158)
Restenosis after previous CEA	34.2% (95/278)	35.9% (52/145)	0.748	36.1% (57/158)
Unfavorable Anatomic Conditions				
Radiation treatment to neck	6.5% (18/278)	6.9% (10/145)	0.840	7.0% (11/158)
Radical neck surgery	2.2% (6/278)	4.8% (7/145)	0.146	3.2% (5/158)
Surgically inaccessible lesions	6.5% (18/278)	9.0% (13/145)	0.432	8.9% (14/158)
Spinal immobility	2.9% (8/278)	6.2% (9/145)	0.119	0.0% (0/158)
Presence of tracheostomy stoma	1.4% (4/278)	2.1% (3/145)	0.695	1.9% (3/158)
Contralateral laryngeal nerve paralysis	0.4% (1/278)	0.7% (1/145)	1.000	0.6% (1/158)

[1]Statistical test of difference between ARCHeR 2 and ARCHeR 3, using Fisher's exact test for categorical values and *t*-test for continuous variables.

TABLE 7.11   Safety Assessment Event Rates of ARCHeR Pivotal Trials (≤30 days)

Event Categories[1]	ARCHeR 2 (N = 278) n	%	ARCHeR 3 (N = 145) n	%	p-Value[2]	ARCHeR 1 (N = 158) n	%
30-Day primary endpoint (death, stroke, MI)	24	8.63	12	8.28	1.000	12	7.59
All stroke, death endpoints	19	6.83	11	7.59	0.842	10	6.33
Death	6	2.16	2	1.38	0.625	3	1.10
Stroke-related	2	0.72	0	0.00	0.406	2	0.74
Not Stroke-related	4	1.44	2	1.38	0.965	0	0.00
Ipsilateral stroke	14	5.04	7	4.83	0.933	6	3.80
Major	3	1.08	2	1.38	0.802	2	1.27
Minor[2]	11	3.96	5	3.45	0.816	4	2.53
Non-ipsilateral stroke	1	0.36	1	0.69	0.653	1	0.63
Non-stroke neurological[3]	6	2.16	1	0.69	0.341	3	1.90

TABLE 7.11 *Continued*

Event Categories[1]	ARCHeR 2 (N = 278)		ARCHeR 3 (N = 145)		p-Value[2]	ARCHeR 1 (N = 158)	
	n	%	n	%		n	%
MI	8	2.88	2	1.38	0.406	4	2.53
Procedural complication	27	9.71	8	5.52	0.194	11	6.96
Hypotension	15	5.40	2	1.38	0.092	6	3.80
Arrhythmia	11	3.96	0	0.00	0.048	5	3.16
Vasospasm	4	1.44	0	0.00	0.238	0	0.00
Dissection	2	0.72	3	2.07	0.223	0	0.00
In-stent thrombosis	1	0.36	1	0.69	0.653	0	0.00
Emergent CEA	2	0.72	0	0.00	0.406	0	0.00
Emergent intervention	1	0.36	1	0.69	0.653	0	0.00
Access site complication[4]	13	4.68	4	2.76	0.405	9	5.70
Requiring repair/ transfusion	8	2.88	2	1.38	0.406	6	3.80
Bleeding[5]	7	2.52	6	4.14	0.387	11	6.96
Requiring transfusion	5	1.80	5	3.45	0.310	9	5.70
GI bleeding	0	0.00	2	1.38	0.015	2	1.27
Adverse events related to device failure or malfunction[6]	2	0.72	1	0.69	1.000	0	0.00

[1]Patients who had multiple events could be counted in more than one category/subcategory of event. Counts represent the number of patients who experienced one or more events.

[2]Two patients suffered strokes that were determined to be nonserious adverse events. However, because the events did not meet the criteria for a serious adverse event (no intervention to prevent permanent impairment, no persistent or significant disability), they are not included in the accounting of serious adverse events. The events are included as strokes in the composite endpoints.

[3]Includes events such as visual/speech disturbances, confusion, seizure, and TIA.

[4]Includes events such as bruising, hematoma, and bleeding.

[5]Includes events such as non–access site bleeding, anemia up to 30 days, and GI bleed up to 30 days.

[6]Three adverse events counted above were categorized as related to device failure/ malfunction.

One dissection in the ARCHeR 2 study was attributed by the physician to the OTW ACCUNET™ System. The physician was not able to cross the lesion with the device. One CEA in the ARCHeR 2 study resulted when the OTW ACCUNET™ System became entangled with the deployed stent and could not be retrieved by the physician.

One emergent intervention in the ARCHeR 3 study resulted when the RX ACCUNET™ filter basket became entangled with the deployed stent and detached from the guide wire during the retrieval attempt. The physician opted to stent the basket in place in the artery. No additional adverse events related to this device malfunction were reported as of the last patient's follow-up (9 months postprocedure).

TABLE 7.12   Efficacy Assessment Event Rates of ARCHeR Pivotal Trial Results

Events	ARCHeR 2 n/N	%	ARCHeR 3 n/N	%	p-Value	ARCHeR 1 n/N	%
One-year primary endpoint (30-day primary endpoint + ipsilateral stroke between 31 and 365 days)[1] [95% confidence interval][2]	10.22% [—, 13.48%]		N/A		N/A	8.28% [—, 12.25%]	
ACCUNET™ device success[3]	264/277	95.3	139/145	95.9	1.000	N/A	
ACCULINK™ device/ procedural success[4]	268/271	98.9	141/142	99.3	1.000	153/156	98.1
Clinical success[5]	249/272	91.5	133/142	93.7	0.562	143/156	91.7
Postprocedure in-lesion minimal lumen diameter							
Mean ± SD (N)	3.64 ± 0.78	(272)	3.79 ± 0.75	(143)	0.064	3.95 ± 0.86	(156)
Range (min, max)	(1.93, 6.89)		(1.93, 6.29)			(1.52, 6.67)	
Postprocedure in-lesion percent diameter stenosis							
Mean ± SD (N)	18.66 ± 11.88	(272)	15.85 ± 12.47	(143)	0.025	20.40 ± 12.38	(156)
Range (min, max)	(0.00, 51.07)		(−12.1, 55.66)			(−12.1, 56.06)	
Target lesion revascularization (clinically indicated)[1,6]			N/A		N/A		
At 6 months	1	0.4				1	0.7
At 12 months	7	2.8				3	2.2
At 24 months	8	3.8				4	3.0
Ultrasound (same or decreased stenosis from baseline exam)			N/A		N/A		
At 6 months	143/196	73.0				84/102	82.4
At 12 months	124/173	71.7				78/97	80.4

[1]Estimated via Kaplan–Meier analysis.

[2]95% one-sided confidence interval by normal approximation, using Peto's formula for the Kaplan–Meier standard error.

[3]Device delivered, placed, and retrieved as described in protocol.

[4]Stent successfully deployed and residual stenosis <50% following stent placement, per core lab reading.

[5]ACCULINK™ device/procedural success in the absence of death, emergency endarterectomy, repeat PTA/thrombolysis of the target vessel, stroke, or MI, within seven days of procedure.

[6]TLR is defined as any repeat invasive procedure, including angioplasty, stenting, endarterectomy or thrombolysis, performed to open or increase the luminal diameter inside or within 10 mm of the previously treated lesion. To be considered clinically indicated, the patient must be symptomatic with ≥50% stenosis or asymptomatic with ≥80% stenosis.

these devices may represent a reduced risk compared to existing technology, the FDA granted expedited review to the ACCULINK™ Carotid Stent System and the RX ACCULINK™ Carotid Stent System.

It seems that the approval of the FDA to the historic control group used in the ARCHeR registries was for the following reasons:

1. The OPC of the historic control was based on multiple landmark studies.
2. Continued update of the OPC was provided by newly published research.
3. The OPC represents the standard of care for this disease.

USE OF ANGIOGRAPHIC LATE LOSS AS PRIMARY ENDPOINT IN DRUG-ELUTING STENT PMA P070015 (XIENCE V DES)[62]

XIENCE V™ (Everolimus Eluting Coronary Stent System)

Study Definitions

- Target lesion revascularization (TLR): Ischemia-driven repeat intervention of the target lesion of the target vessel.
- Target vessel revascularization (TVR): Ischemia-driven repeat intervention (PCI or CABG) of the target vessel.
- Target vessel failure (TVF): Composite of TVR, cardiac death, and MI.
- Major adverse cardiac events (MACE): Composite of cardiac death, MI, and TLR by CABG or PCI.

Late Lumen Loss (LL)

- Difference between the postprocedure MLD and MLD at follow-up angiography.
- In-segment versus in-stent.
- Angiographic binary restenosis (ABR).
- Angiographic follow-up % diameter stenosis of ≥50%.
- Percent diameter stenosis (%DS).
- Calculated as $100 * (1 - MLD/RVD)$ using the mean values from two orthogonal views (when possible) by QCA.

The *analysis lesion* is defined as the target lesion for subjects with a single de novo lesion and a randomly selected lesion for subjects with two de novo lesions. If the randomized analysis lesion could not be treated for any reason, the other target lesion, by default, became the analysis lesion.

Stent Thrombosis Levels of Evidence

Definite/Confirmed   Acute coronary syndrome was complicated by:

- Angiographic confirmation of thrombus or occlusion *OR*
- Pathologic confirmation of acute thrombosis.

Probable

- Unexplained death within 30 days.
- Target vessel MI without angiographic confirmation of thrombosis or other identified culprit lesion.

Possible   Death was unexplained after 30 days.

Key Inclusion Criteria

- Evidence of myocardial ischemia (e.g., angina, silent ischemia, positive functional study or a reversible changes in the ECG consistent with ischemia).
- Target lesion(s) in a major artery or branch with a visually estimated stenosis of ≥50% and <100% with a TIMI flow of ≥1.
- Target lesion length:
    - ≤28 mm in length by visual estimation (SPIRIT II & III).
    - ≤12 mm (SPIRIT FIRST).
- Target vessel reference diameter:
    - ≥2.5 mm and ≤3.75 mm (SPIRIT III).
    - >3.75 mm and ≤4.25 mm (SPIRIT III 4.0-mm arm).
    - ≥2.5 mm and ≤4.25 mm (SPIRIT II).
    - 3.0 mm only (SPIRIT FIRST).

Pivotal US Trial

- Randomized (2:1), single-blind, noninferiority trial in 1002 subjects.

- Evaluation of the XIENCE V compared to TAXUS in the treatment of up to two de novo lesions ≤28 mm in length in native coronary arteries with RVD ≥2.5 mm to ≤3.75 mm.
- Two co-primary endpoints:
  In-segment late loss (LL) at 240 days (one-sided alpha of 0.025 and a difference of in-segment late loss between the XIENCE V and TAXUS arms of no more than 0.195 mm).
  Ischemia-driven target vessel failure (TVF) at 270 days (one-sided alpha of 0.05 and a difference in TVF rate of no more than 5.5%).

Important Secondary Endpoints

- TVF, TLR, and MACE at 30, 180, 270 days, and 1, 2, 3, 4, and 5 years.
- Persisting incomplete stent apposition, late-acquired incomplete stent apposition, and thrombosis at 240 days.
- Acute success (clinical device and clinical procedure).
- Proximal, distal, and in-stent LL at 240 days.
- In-stent and in-segment percent diameter stenosis (%DS) and percent angiographic binary restenosis (% ABR) rate at 240 days.
- In-stent percent volume obstruction (%VO) at 240 days.

Figure 7.2 shows the SPIRIT III trial design where 668 and 334 patients were randomized (in 2:1 ratio) to the XIENE V and TAXUS arms, respectively.

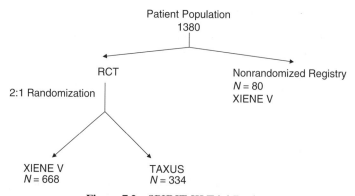

Figure 7.2 SPIRIT III Trial Design

SPIRIT III (RCT) Statistical Analysis

- Primary endpoint: 240-day in-segment late loss (LL).
- Noninferiority hypotheses:

    H_0: In-segment LL XIENCE V – In-segment LL TAXUS $\geq \delta$.

    H_A: In-segment LL XIENCE V – In-segment LL TAXUS $< \delta$, where $\delta = 0.195$.

    A sample size of 338 in XIENCE V and 169 in TAXUS will have a power of 99% at one-sided alpha level of 0.025.

- Superiority hypotheses:

    H_0: In-segment LL XIENCE V $\geq$ In-segment LL TAXUS.

    H_A: In-segment LL XIENCE V $<$ In-segment LL TAXUS at two-sided alpha level of 0.05.

- Co-primary endpoint: 270-day ischemia-driven target vessel failure (TVF).
- Noninferiority Hypotheses:

    H_0: TVF XIENCE V – TVF TAXUS $\geq 5.5\%$.

    H_A: TVF XIENCE V – TVF TAXUS $< 5.5\%$.

    A sample size of 660 in XIENCE V and 330 in TAXUS will have a power of 89% at one-sided alpha level of 0.05.

- Superiority hypotheses:

    H_0: TVF XIENCE V $\geq$ TVF TAXUS.

    H_A: TVF XIENCE V $<$ TVF TAXUS at two-sided alpha level of 0.05.

Baseline patients demographic/clinical characteristics and baseline lesion characteristics in the SPIRIRT III RCT are shown in Tables 7.13 and 7.14.

Procedural Success and 30-Day MACE   Major adverse cardiac events that presented in the first 30 days were reversed by:

- Clinical device success (per lesion).
- XIENCE 98.3% versus TAXUS 98.7%.
- Clinical procedure success (per subject).
- XIENCE 98.5% versus TAXUS 97.3%.

The 30-day rates of MACE and MI are presented in Table 7.15. The results of the primary endpoint, 240 day in segment late loss, are shown

TABLE 7.13   Baseline Demographic and Clinical Characteristics

	XIENCE V (*N* = 669)	TAXUS (*N* = 333)
Age (yrs)	63.23 ± 10.53 (669)	62.80 ± 10.24 (332)
Male	70.1% (469/669)	65.7% (218/332)
Current cigarette use	23.4% (154/659)	22.5% (73/324)
Any diabetes	29.6% (198/669)	27.9% (92/330)
Diabetes requiring insulin	7.8% (52/669)	5.5% (18/330)
Hypertension requiring medication	76.2% (510/669)	74.0% (245/331)
Hyperlipidemia requiring medication	74.2% (489/659)	71.5% (233/326)
Prior myocardial infarction	19.9% (130/652)	18.0% (59/327)
Prior PCI	26.3% (175/666)	27.7% (92/332)
Prior CABG	8.56% (57/666)	3.61% (12/332)
Stable angina	53.3% (350/657)	47.7% (156/327)
Unstable angina	18.7% (123/657)	25.1% (82/327)

TABLE 7.14   Baseline Lesion and Vessel Characteristics

	XIENCE V (*N* = 669)	TAXUS (*N* = 333)
Number of Lesions/Vessels Treated		
One	84.6% (566/669)	84.6% (281/332)
Two	15.4% (103/669)	15.4% (51/332)
Target Lesion(S)		
RVD, mm	2.77 ± 0.45 (767)	2.76 ± 0.46 (382)
Lesion length, mm	14.70 ± 5.59 (767)	14.73 ± 5.70 (379)
Preprocedure % diameter stenosis	69.96 ± 13.34 (767)	69.44 ± 13.62 (382)
Vessel Location		
LAD	41.3% (317/768)	42.9% (164/382)
LCX	25.5% (196/768)	26.2% (100/382)
RCA	31.0% (238/768)	28.5% (109/382)
Postprocedure % Diameter Stenosis		
In-stent	0.33 ± 8.93 (762)	−0.22 ± 9.94 (379)
In-segment	13.54 ± 7.58 (765)	14.40 ± 7.10 (379)

TABLE 7.15   MACE and MI Rates at 30 Days

	XIENCE (*N* = 669)	TAXUS (*N* = 333)
MACE	1.2%	2.4%
Q-Wave MI	0.0%	0.0%
Non–Q-wave MI	0.9%	2.1%

TABLE 7.16   Primary Endpoint Results

	XIENCE V (N = 376)	TAXUS (N = 188)	Difference [95%, CI]	Noninferior p-Value[a]
At 240 day in segment, late loss (mm)	014 ± 0.41 (301)	0.28 ± 0.48 (134)	−0.14 [−0.23, −0.05)	<0.0001

[a]One-sided noninferiority test using asymptotic test statistic with noninferiority margin of 0.195 mm, compared at a 0.025 significance level.

TABLE 7.17   Rate of Target Vessel Failure at 9 Months

	XIENCE V (N = 669)	TAXUS (N = 333)	Difference [95% CI]	Noninferior p-Value[a]
Faiture rate at 9 months	7.6% (50/657)	9.7% (31/320)	−2.08% [−5.90%, 1.75%]	<0.0001

[a]One-sided noninferiority test using asymptotic test statistic with noninferiority margin of 5.5%, to be compared at a 0.05 significance level.

TABLE 7.18   Clinical Outcome at 9 to 12 Months

	XIENCE V (N = 669)	TAXUS (N = 333)
Death	1.2%	0.9%
Cardiac death	0.6%	0.6%
MI	2.3%	3.1%
TLR	2.7%	5.0%
Non-TL TVR	2.9%	4.1%
TVF	7.6%	9.7%

in Table 7.16. The nine-month rate of target vessel failure (TVF) is shown in Table 7.17. As shown in Tables 7.16 and 7.17 both co-primary endpoints met.

Tables 7.18 and 7.19 list the clinical outcomes at 9-month and the 12-month stent thrombosis. Table 7.20 shows other angiographic results at 8 months, such as, in stent late loss, in-stent %DS, in-segment %DS, in-stent ABR, and in-segment ABR. The IVUS results at 8 months are shown Table 7.21. The data for patients with complete assessment of angiographic data at 8 months is shown in Table 7.22. One subject did not provide written informed consent and was inadvertently randomized into TAXUS RCT. Data from this subject is excluded from all data analyses.

TABLE 7.19   Stent Thrombosis at 12 Months

	XIENCE V ($N = 669$)	TAXUS ($N = 333$)
Stent Thrombosis (Per Protocol)		
Acute (1 day)	0.1% (1/669)	0.0% (0/330)
Sub-acute (1 to 30 days)	0.3% (2/667)	0.0% (0/330)
Late (31 to 393 days)	0.3% (2/646)	0.6% (2/317)
Total	0.8% (5/647)	0.6% (2/317)
Stent Thrombosis (Per ARC Definite + Probable; TLR not Censored)		
Acute (1 day)	0.1% (1/669)	0.0% (0/330)
Sub-acute (1 to 30 days)	0.4% (3/667)	0.0% (0/330)
Late (30 to 393 days)	0.5% (3/651)	0.6% (2/319)
Total	1.1% (7/648)	0.6% (2/317)
[95% CI]	[0.44%, 2.21%]	[0.08%, 2.26%]

TABLE 7.20   Other Angiographic Results at 8 Months

	XIENCE V ($N = 669$, $M = 772$)	TAXUS ($N = 333$, $M = 383$)	Difference [95% CI]
In-stent late loss, mm	(342) 0.16 ± 0.41	(158) 0.30 ± 0.53	−0.15 [−0.24, −0.05]
In-stent %DS	(343) 5.92 ± 16.40	(158) 10.30 ± 21.43	−4.38 [−8.16, −0.60]
In-segment %DS	(344) 18.77 ± 14.43	(158) 22.82 ± 16.35	−4.05 [−7.03, −1.06]
In-stent ABR	2.3% (8/343)	5.7% (9/158)	−3.36% [−7.32%, 0.59%]
In-segment ABR	4.7% (16/344)	8.9% (14/158)	−4.21% [−9.17%, 0.75%]

Note: N is the total number of subjects; M is the total number of lesions.

TABLE 7.21   Other IVUS Results at 8 Months

	XIENCE V ($N = 669$, $M = 772$)	TAXUS ($N = 333$, $M = 383$)
NIH volume, mm	310.13 ± 11.46 (101)	20.87 ± 31.51 (41)
%VO	6.91 ± 6.35 (98)	11.21 ± 9.86 (39)
Incomplete Apposition		
Postprocedure	34.4% (31/90)	25.6% (11/43)
At 240 days	25.6% (23/90)	16.3% (7/43)
Persisting	24.4% (22/90)	14.0% (6/43)
Late acquired	1.1% (1/90)	2.3% (1/43)

Note: N is the total number of subjects; M is the total number of lesions.

TABLE 7.22   **Missing Angiographic Data in SPIRITIII (RCT)**

	XIENCE V ($N = 376$)	TAXUS ($N = 188$)
Completers	80.1% (301/376)	71.7% (134/187)

Summary of SPIRIT III RCT

- The SPIRIT III RCT successfully met both of its co-primary end-points by demonstrating noninferiority of XIENCE V to TAXUS with respect to 240-day in-segment late loss and 270 day target vessel failure (TVF).
- Angiographic and IVUS results suggest a consistent trend toward lower restenosis in XIENCE V compared with TAXUS.
- The Xience V stent had comparable safety outcomes out to 12 months compared with TAXUS.

Key Limitations

- As in many experimental studies, SPIRIT III was not designed to establish safety and efficacy in specific patient subgroups or any secondary clinical endpoints.
- Post hoc data analyses and apparent trends toward significance need to be interpreted cautiously when assessing performance in specific patient subgroups or across multiple secondary endpoints.
- At 37 sites overall, 199 subjects (140 XIENCE V and 59 TAXUS subjects) were evaluated by unblinded study personnel at nine-month follow-up visit, representing nearly 20% (199/1002) of the total SPIRIT III RCT cohort. Subjects that were evaluated by unblinded study personnel were excluded and did not alter the study outcome.
- Evaluable angiographic data were available for 77% of the subjects randomized to receive eight-month angiography for analysis of a co-primary endpoint of in-segment late loss.

SPIRIT III 4.0-mm Arm

The SPIRIT III 4.0-mm arm was a single-arm, nonrandomized, prospective, multicenter study.

Objective   The study was designed to evaluate XIENCE V compared with TAXUS in the treatment of up to two de novo lesions ≤28 mm in length in native coronary arteries with the RVD >3.75 mm to ≤4.25 mm.

Primary Endpoint

- In-segment late loss at 240 days in the 4.0-mm XIENCE V arm was compared with that of the TAXUS arm from the RCT with a non-inferiority margin (delta) of 0.195 mm.
- The interim analysis was conducted on the first 69 subjects enrolled (after unblinding of the RCT) with an adjusted *p*-value (decision boundary) applied to the analysis of in-segment late loss.

Baseline patients demographic/clinical characteristics and baseline lesion characteristics in the SPIRIT III 4.0-mm arm are shown in Tables 7.23 and 7.24.

Procedural Success and 30-Day MACE   The 30-day rate of MACE in the SPIRIT III 4.0-mm arm is shown in Table 7.25.

- Clinical device success (per lesion)
- XIENCE 4.0 mm 98.5% versus TAXUS 98.7% versus XIENCE RCT 98.3%

TABLE 7.23   Baseline Demographic and Clinical Characteristics

	XIENCE V 4.0 mm (*N* = 69)
Age (yrs)	61.93 ± 11.20 (69)
Male	72.5% (50/69)
Current cigarette use	27.9% (19/68)
Any diabetes	30.4% (21/69)
Diabetes requiring insulin	8.7% (6/69)
Hypertension requiring medication	65.2% (45/69)
Hyperlipidemia requiring medication	77.9% (53/68)
Prior myocardial infarction	17.4% (12/69)
Prior PCI	18.8% (13/69)
Prior CABG	5.8% (4/69)
Stable angina	47.8% (32/67)
Unstable angina	19.4% (13/67)

TABLE 7.24   Baseline Lesion and Vessel Characteristics

	XIENCE V 4.0-mm Arm (N = 69, M = 69)	TAXUS RCT (N = 188, M = 220)	XIENCE V RCT (N = 376, M = 427)
Target Vessel			
LAD	26.1% (18/69)	43.6% (96/220)	40.5% (173/427)
Circumflex or ramus	17.4% (12/69)	28.6% (63/220)	27.9% (119/427)
RCA	56.5% (39/69)	27.7% (61/220)	31.6% (135/427)
LMCA	0.0% (0/69)	0.0% (0/220)	0.0% (0/427)
Pre-procedure RVD (mm) Mean ± SD (m)	3.53 ± 0.36 (69)	2.77 ± 0.46 (220)	2.75 ± 0.44 (427)
Pre-procedure %DS Mean ± SD (m)	71.37 ± 13.38 (69)	70.33 ± 13.48 (220)	70.41 ± 13.32 (427)
Lesion length (mm) Mean ± SD (m)	15.43 ± 6.21 (69)	14.99 ± 5.88 (218)	14.92 ± 5.73 (427)

Note: N is the total number of subjects; M is the total number of lesions.

TABLE 7.25   MACE in the SPIRITIII 4.0-mm Arm at 30 Days

	XIENCE V 4.0 mm (N = 69)	TAXUS RCT (N = 333)
MACE	4.3%	2.4%
Q-wave MI	0.0%	0.0%
Non–Q-wave MI	4.3%	2.1%

- Clinical procedure success (per subject)
- XIENCE 4.0 mm 94.2% versus TAXUS 97.3% versus XIENCE RCT 98.5%
- 30-Day MACE

Data for the SPIRIT III 4.0 arm are presented in Tables 7.19 through 7.22. The 30-day rates of MACE and MI are presented in Table 7.19. The primary endpoint result is presented in Table 7.26. The angiographic results at 8 months and the clinical outcomes at 9 to 12 months are presented in Tables 7.27 and 7.28.

The results of the primary endpoint, 240-day in segment late loss is shown in Table 7.26. These results indicate that the primary endpoint was met.

TABLE 7.26 Primary Endpoint Results

	XIENCE V 4.0-mm Arm ($N = 69$)	TAXUS RCT ($N = 188$)	"Noninferiority" p-Value[a]
240-day in-segment late loss Mean ± SD (n)	0.17 ± 0.38 (49)	0.28 ± 0.48 (134)	<0.0001

[a]One-sided by noninferiority test using asymptotic test statistic with noninferiority margin of 0.195 mm, compared at a 0.0377 significance level.

TABLE 7.27 Angiography Results at 8 Months

	XIENCE V 4.0-mm Arm ($N = 69$, $M = 69$)	TAXUS RCT ($N = 188$, $M = 220$)	XIENCE V RCT ($N = 376$, $M = 427$)
Pre-procedure RVD (mm) Mean ± SD (m)	3.53 ± 0.36 (69)	2.77 ± 0.46 (220)	2.75 ± 0.44 (427)
Pre-procedure (%) Diameter stenosis (% DS) Mean ± SD (m)	71.37 ± 13.38 (69)	70.33 ± 13.48 (220)	70.41 ± 13.32 (427)
240-Day in-segment (%DS) Mean ± SD (m)	17.92 ± 10.83 (49)	22.82 ± 16.35 (158)	18.77 ± 14.43 (344)
In-stent late loss (mm) Mean ± SD (m)	0.12 ± 0.34 (49)	0.30 ± 0.53 (158)	0.16 ± 0.41 (342)
240-Day in-segment Angiographic binary Restenosis (ABR)	2.0 % (1/49)	8.9% (14/158)	4.7% (16/344)

Note: N is the total number of subjects; M is the total number of lesions.

TABLE 7.28 Clinical Outcome at 9 to 12 Months

	XIENCE V 4.0 mm ($N = 69$)
Cardiac death	1.5%
Non–Q-wave MI	4.4%
Q-Wave MI	0.0%
TLR	1.5%
Non–TL TVR	0.0%
TVF	5.9%

Summary of SPIRIT III 4.0-mm Registry Arm

- The SPIRIT III 4.0-mm arm successfully met its primary endpoint of 240-day in-segment late loss.
- The secondary angiographic endpoints demonstrated lower observed rates of restenosis compared to the TAXUS control and were also similar to XIENCE V data from the SPIRIT III RCT.
- The SPIRIT III 4.0-mm arm was not designed to adequately evaluate clinical outcomes, but for the subjects available for clinical analysis. The results of the XIENCE V 4.0 mm were comparable to those seen in the SPIRIT III RCT.

Key Limitations The SPIRIT III 4.0-mm arm was nonrandomized. So an interpretation of the results needs to take into account the following:

- The primary analysis was not adjusted for covariates in this non-randomized study.
- TAXUS does not have approved 4.0-mm drug-eluting stent.
- TAXUS is not indicated for the treatment of RVD >3.75 mm, whereas XIENCE V 4.0 mm is intended for the treatment of RVD between 3.75 and 4.25 mm.
- Only 71% (49/69) of enrolled subjects had qualifying follow-up angiograms.
- The study was not to designed to evaluate clinical endpoints, but to establish the effectiveness of the 4.0-mm platform by demonstrating comparability of in-segment late loss to TAXUS in the SPIRIT III RCT.

FDA Panel Decision The Circulatory System Devices Advisory panel to the FDA recommended approval for the XIENCE V Everolimus Eluting Coronary Stent System. The FDA advisory committee recommended the XIENCE V stent system for approval provided that conditions be met related to a postmarketing study and language added about the dual antiplatelet therapy. These conditions were followed, and the FDA approved the XIENCE V coronary stent system.

Bioethics in Clinical Research

Bioethics for clinical trials were developed after World War II when Nazi regime crimes were discovered in the medical field. The standards of ethical clinical research are detailed in:

- The International Conference of Harmonization (ICH)
- The Declaration of Helsinki
- The National Research Act
- The Belmont Report

The responsibilities of sponsor and investigator are based on the concept of good clinical practice (GCP), as expressed in the International Conference on Harmonization (ICH). GCP standards were developed to help investigators perform clinical trials in a way that ensures the safety of trial subjects and confidentiality of their medical records. GCP provides guidance on the design, conduct, monitoring, auditing, recording, analysis, and reporting of clinical trials, and for posterity provides assurance that the data and reported results are credible and accurate, and that the rights, integrity, and confidentiality of trial subjects were protected.

The protection of human subjects is usually done systematically through:

The Design and Management of Medical Device Clinical Trials: Strategies and Challenges, by Salah Abdel-aleem
Copyright © 2010 John Wiley & Sons, Inc.

- Monitoring by the IRB.
- Risk/benefit assessment of each trial.
- Consideration for the safety and privacy of the trial subjects.
- Maintenance of confidentiality of regarding trial data.

An essential ethical condition for a clinical trial comparing two treatments for a disease is that there be no good reason for thinking one is better than the other. Usually the investigators expect the new treatment to be better, but there should not be solid evidence one way or the other until proved.

Protecting the rights, interests, and safety of research subjects must continue for the study's duration. Observing the ethical standards of a clinical trial subject is the responsibility of several groups, including research the institutional review board/ethics committees, investigators and their research staffs, and sponsors. This chapter describes the ethical standards established by law that ensure adequate protection of the rights and welfare of human subjects. The chapter also discusses the challenges associated with the bioethical nature of most clinical trials, for example, the basic ethical principles and their origins and the challenges clinical trials pose to the IRB/EC.

BIOETHICAL CHALLENGES IN CLINICAL STUDIES

Principles of GCP Guidance

The main objectives of GCP guidance can be summarized as follows:

1. Clinical trials should be conducted in accordance with the ethical principles expressed in the Declaration of Helsinki, and the Belmont Report as are consistent with GCP and the applicable regulatory requirements.
2. Before a trial is initiated, foreseeable risks and inconveniences should be weighed against the anticipated benefit for the individual trial subject and society. A trial should be initiated and continued only if the anticipated benefits justify the risks.
3. The rights, safety, and well-being of the trial subjects are the most important considerations and should prevail over interests of science and society.
4. The available nonclinical and clinical information on an investigational product should be adequate to support the proposed clinical trial.

5. Clinical trials should be scientifically sound, and the protocol described in a clear language.

6. A trial should be conducted in compliance with the protocol that has received prior institutional review board (IRB)/independent ethics committee (IEC) approval/favorable opinion.

7. The medical care given to, and medical decisions made on behalf of, subjects should always be the responsibility of a qualified physician or, when appropriate, of a qualified dentist.

8. Each individual involved in conducting a trial should be qualified by education, training, and experience to perform his or her respective tasks.

9. Freely given informed consent should be obtained from every subject prior to clinical trial participation.

10. All clinical trial information should be recorded, handled, and stored in a way that allows its accurate reporting, interpretation, and verification.

11. The confidentiality of records that could identify subjects should be protected, respecting the privacy and confidentiality rules in accordance with the applicable regulatory requirements.

12. Investigational products should be manufactured, handled, and stored in accordance with applicable good manufacturing practice (GMP). They should be used in accordance with the approved protocol.

13. Systems with procedures that ensure the quality of every aspect of the trial should be implemented.

Beyond these thirteen principles, GCPs address the key components of clinical trials, including:

- Institutional Review Boards (IRBs)
- Investigators
- Sponsors
- Protocols and protocol amendments
- Investigator's brochure
- Essential documents

GOOD CLINICAL PRACTICE FOR THE INVESTIGATOR

Clinical trials are designed, implemented, conducted and reported using good clinical practices (GCPs) to give public assurance that data are complete, correct, and accurate and that the rights, welfare, and confidentiality of subjects are protected.

GCP for the Investigator includes:

- **Direct responsibility.** The study investigator is responsible for supervising the entire study, research staff, medical management of the subject, and obtaining consent of the study subject. The study investigator should be also familiar with IRB regulations and reporting procedures, and thus conduct the study in accordance with clinical protocol.
- **Staff and facilities.** The clinical site should have the adequate staff and facilities. The facility should be equipped with the required labs as requested for the study, as well as adequate storage area for the product and study documents. There should also be adequate area for study monitors.
- **Medical management of subject.** The principal investigator (PI) supervises use of medical drugs and devices but can delegate some of these responsibilities to the staff.
- **IRB.** The PI should be familiar with his/her IRB regulation, and reporting procedures for adverse events, protocol deviations, and so forth.
- **Protocol compliance.** The PI should conduct the study in accordance with the study protocol.
- **Informed consent.** The PI is responsible for obtaining consent from every study subject, unless a waiver of consenting subjects is obtained from FDA.
- **Records, reports, source documents.** The PI should keep all records, reports, and source documents of the study in accordance to the time period specified in the protocol.
- **Events AE/SAE.** The PI should report all AE, SAE in accordance with the clinical protocol.
- **Financial disclosure.** The PI should provide a financial disclosure certificate to the sponsor stating all his/her financial assets in the company.

WHO PRINCIPLES OF GCP

The principles of WHO on bioethical conduct of clinical trials follow:

Principle 1 The basic ethic of respect for persons, of beneficence and justice, must be protected. Respect for persons is implemented by treating the trial subject as autonomous agent who is be entitled to full protection of the law. Beneficence is implemented by maximizing benefits and minimizing harm to subject and carefully assessing the risks/benefits analysis of the study. Justice is implemented by using fair criteria for selecting subjects for the study, such as by randomization.

Principle 2 Research involving humans should be scientifically justified and described in a protocol.

Principle 3 Foreseeable risks and discomforts and any anticipated benefit(s) for the individual trial subject and society should be identified.

Principle 4 The anticipated benefit(s) for the individual research subject and society clearly outweigh the risks.

Principle 5 Research involving humans should receive independent ethics committee/institutional review board (IEC/IRB) approval/favorable opinion prior to initiation.

Principle 6 Research involving humans should be conducted in compliance with the approved protocol.

Principle 7 Freely given informed consent should be obtained from every subject prior to research participation in accordance with national culture(s) and requirements. When a subject is not capable of giving informed consent, the permission of a legally authorized representative should be obtained in accordance with applicable law.

Principle 8 Medical personnel who are qualified by education, training, and experience should be responsible for the medical care of trial subjects, and for any medical decision(s) made on their behalf.

Principle 9 All clinical trial information should be recorded, handled, and stored in a way that allows its accurate reporting, interpretation, and verification.

Principle 10 The confidentiality of records that could identify subjects should be protected.

Principle 11 Investigational products should be manufactured, handled, and stored in accordance with applicable good manufacturing practices.

Principle 12 Quality assurance of every aspect of the trial should be implemented.

GUIDELINES AND ETHICAL PRINCIPLES

The founding guidelines and ethical principles for the protection of human subjects in research today were provided by the Nuremberg Code (1947), the Declaration of Helsiniki (1964), the National Research Act (1974), and the Belmont Report (1979).

Nuremberg Code, 1947

The Nuremberg Code was drafted as a set of standards for judging physicians and scientists who had conducted biomedical experiments on concentration camp prisoners. The Nuremberg Code's three basic tenets are (1) voluntary consent, (2) benefits outweigh risks, and (3) ability of the subject to terminate participation. Essentially informed consent, as defined in the Nuremberg Code, was the first legal attempt to deal with ethical issues of research and so became the prototype of many later codes. As biomedical research advanced, international need for a more specific code of ethics led to, the formulation of the Declaration of Helsinki.

Declaration of Helsinki

The Declaration of Helsinki consists of recommendations for medical doctors involved in biomedical research with human subjects. It was adopted by the 18th World Medical Assembly held in Helsinki, Finland, in 1964, and revised in 1975, 1983, 1989, and 1996. The Declaration of Helsinki has put forward general guidance on ethical conduct of biomedical research using human subjects.

National Research Act, 1974

The National Research Act established the National Commission for the Protection of Human Subjects of Biomedical and Behavioral Research. This Commission has required institutions receiving HEW support for human subjects research to maintain review boards (TRBs). HEW, an acronym for the Department of Health, Education and Welfare, was created under President Eisenhower, when the Department of Education Organization Act was signed into law, providing for a separate Department of Education.

The Belmont Report

The Belmont Report covers ethical principles and provides guidelines for the protection of human subjects of research. This critical report was prepared by the National Commission for the Protection of Human Subjects of Biomedical and Behavioral Research on April 18, 1979. The Belmont Report considers three ethical principles to be basic to the protection of human subjects: (1) respect for persons-individual autonomy, including protection of individuals with reduced autonomy (by informed consent); (2) beneficence-maximized benefits and minimized harms; and (3) justice-equitable distribution of research costs and benefits (for the groups of people bearing the burden of the research).

Federal Regulations and Policy

45 CFR 46 represents the basic US Department of Health and Human Services policy for protection of human research subjects. The HHS policy was adopted in May 1974 and was revised January 13, 1984, and again on June 18, 1991. 45 CFR 46 has four parts (commonly referred to as Subparts A–D). Subpart A (Federal Policy for the Protection of Human Subjects—or "The Common Rule") is the heart of federal regulation and policy. It is adopted by all federal funding agencies, so it is known as the Common Rule.

The federal regulations of 45 CFR 46 contain three basic protections for human subjects: (1) institutional assurances, (2) IRB review, and (3) informed consent. Federal Policy 45 CFR 46 defines IRB function and operations, establishes criteria for exemption status, determines categories for expedited review, and classifies vulnerable populations.

IRB Structure

Under federal regulations, the IRB must be a diverse group in terms of gender and racial background. Specifically, the IRB must consist of:

- At least five members of varying backgrounds who are sufficiently qualified, not solely of one profession, and gender diversity.
- At least one nonscientist.
- At least one member not affiliated with Institution.
- Expertise on "vulnerable populations" (prisoners, children, pregnant women, etc.).
- Outside consultants.

The main responsibilities of an IRB are to:

- Review and approve, require modifications, or disapprove all research.

- Require that Informed consent be in accordance with regulations.
- Require documentation of informed consent or opt to waive documentation in accordance with regulations.
- Notify investigators, in writing, of decisions.
- Conduct continuing review of research no less than once a year.

IRB REVIEW PROCESS

Exempt review, full review, and expedited review are three possible mechanisms by which initial research proposals involving human subjects are reviewed. Institution-specific determinations on the method by which applications will be reviewed (when, by whom, how, etc.) usually are set forth in an institution's Federal-wide Assurance (FWA) application. With respect to expedited review procedures, generally, protocols that are reviewed via an expedited process are evaluated by the same ethical standards and must meet the same approval criteria as those that receive full IRB review. However, the review process may not require discussion at a convened IRB meeting. According to federal guidelines, an expedited review procedure consists of a review of research involving human subjects by the IRB chairperson or by one or more experienced reviewers designated by the chairperson from among members of the IRB in accordance with the requirements set forth in 45 CFR 46.

Following is a brief description of each type of review. Possible outcomes of initial review, criteria for IRB approval, kinds of risk, evaluation of risk, and the protection of privacy and confidentiality are important components of the full review. A brief introduction to continuing review is also provided.

Exempt Review

Some research is "exempt" from federal regulations, but the IRB of the Institution (*not* the investigator) must certify this. Generally, in the Federal-wide Assurance (FWA) filed with OHRP, the IRB sets up the conditions under which research may be reviewed as "exempt." Thus it is up to the individual IRB to determine the exempt research to be carried out by its institution. The following kinds of research with human subjects may qualify for exemption:

- Research using existing data, documents, records, specimens, (pathological or diagnostic) if publicly available or unidentifiable.

- Research on elected or appointed public officials or candidates for public office.
- Evaluation of public benefit service programs.
- Taste and food quality evaluation and consumer acceptance studies.
- Normal educational practices.
- Educational tests, surveys, interviews, or observation of public behavior unless identified and sensitive.

It is important to note that research is considered *not* exempt if the following are involved:

- Human subjects if identified *and* disclosed could place subjects at risk.
- Pregnant women.
- Fetuses and neonates.
- Human in vitro fertilization.
- Prisoners.
- Minors in survey/interview research.
- Observation of minor if researcher is a participant observer.

Expedited Review

Research is considered for expedited review if the following applies:

- Presents no more than minimal risk to participants.
- Does not involve certain vulnerable populations, namely, prisoners, persons over whom the researcher is in a position of authority, and the mentally disabled.

It is important to note that continuing review of research that meets these criteria may also be conducted via an expedited process. Generally, continuing review is appropriate to the degree of potential risk and is conducted not less than once a year. This type of review is briefly summarized in the next subsection on the full IRB review.

Full IRB Review

All research that is not exempt and does not meet the criteria for expedited review is reviewed via a full IRB review, at a regularly convened meeting in which a majority of members are present, at least one nonscientist is present, and approval is determined by the majority of those present. Members with a conflict of interest must be absent during discussion and vote. Further, should the quorum fail during a meeting (e.g., those with conflicts being excused, loss of a nonscientist, or early departures), no further votes can be taken unless the quorum can be restored.

Generally, criteria for IRB approval is based on the ethical standards and guidelines outlined in the Belmont Report, specifically:

- Risks to subjects are minimized.
- Risks are reasonable in relation to anticipated benefits.
- Selection of subjects is equitable.
- Informed consent is sought from each subject.
- Informed consent is appropriately documented.
- When appropriate, (1) data collection is monitored to ensure subject safety, (2) privacy and confidentiality of subjects are protected, and (3) additional safeguards are included for vulnerable populations.

The IRB very carefully examines the kinds of risk posed by research. Specifically, risks can be categorized into three categories: (1) participant risks (i.e., physical, psychological, social/emotional, legal), (2) investigator risks, and (3) societal risks. It is important to recognize that the IRB's evaluation of risk is based on the "minimal risk" standard, which indicates that the probability and magnitude of harm or discomfort anticipated in the research must not exceed that ordinarily encountered in daily life. Based on this ethically and federally mandated standard, the IRB must in its evaluation of risk:

- Identify the risks associated with the research.
- Determine that the risks will be minimized as much as possible.
- Identify the probable benefits to be derived from the research to subjects and society.
- Determine that the risks are reasonable in relation to benefits to subjects (i.e., risk/benefit ratio; refer to the Belmont Report for an introduction to this concept).
- Ensure that potential subjects will be provided with an accurate and fair description of the risks and benefits.

- Determine intervals of periodic review (i.e., continuing review at least once a year).

As a rule of thumb, investigators should thoughtfully consider the kinds of risk their research poses and not merely guess or assume that there is no risk. This is critical because OHRP does not make determinations based on inadequate information. Thus investigators must look at their research procedures to determine risk, consider vulnerability of participants, and take steps to minimize risk of harm to subjects. For example, a social psychologist studying date rape in young women must minimize the risk of emotional distress to these women by providing referrals to appropriate treatment services.

Investigators should also be aware of three key definitions pertaining to the protection of privacy and confidentiality of participants. First, "privacy" refers to a person's right to control access to information about him/herself. Second, "confidentiality" pertains to the right to keep private information from being divulged in the course of research. Third, the concept of "anonymity" refers to the process of record keeping whereby no names or identifying information can link subjects to the data. Investigators generally do maintain confidentiality and anonymity by using a coding system to disguise or cleanse data of any identifying information, but as an additional practice, they should carefully store any identifying information in a secure, limited-access location.

An important process available to investigators that should not be overlooked is the "Certificate of Confidentiality" for extremely sensitive information. The certificate is issued by the federal government in special circumstances to protect the "privacy" of research subjects and protect investigators against the "compelled disclosure of identifying information about subjects of biomedical, behavioral, clinical, and other research." Stated differently, it protects investigators from being forced to reveal the identity of participants in their research project in legal proceedings. A research project is considered sensitive if it involves any of the following:

- Information relating to sexual attitudes, preferences, or practices.
- Information relating to the use of alcohol, drugs, or other additive products.
- Information pertaining to illegal conduct.
- Information that, if released, could reasonably be damaging to an individual's financial standing, employability, or reputation within the community.

- Information that would normally be recorded in a patient's medical record, and the disclosure of which could reasonably lead to a social stigmatization of discrimination.
- Information pertaining to an individual's psychological well-being or mental health.
- Genetic information.

Absolute risk difference The difference in size of risk between two groups. For example, if one group has a 15% risk of contracting a particular disease, and the other has a 10% risk of getting the disease, the risk difference is five percentage points.

Adverse effect An adverse event for which the causal relation between the drug/intervention and the event is at least a reasonable possibility. The term adverse effect applies to all interventions.

Adverse event An adverse outcome that occurs during or after the use of a drug or other intervention but is not necessarily caused by the drug or intervention.

Authorized representative An authorized representative is an entity explicitly designated by a manufacturer to act on his or her behalf in carrying out certain tasks in Europe. An authorized representative must be established within.

CE French abbreviation for *Conformité Européene*.

CE logo The "CE" marking is a manufacturer's attestation that a product complies with all applicable European directive and essential requirements.

Confidence interval (CI) A measure of the uncertainty around the main finding of a statistical estimates of unknown quantities, such as the odds ratio comparing an experimental intervention with a control, are usually presented as a point estimate and a 95% confidence interval. This means that if someone were to keep repeating a study in other samples from the same population, 95% of the confidence intervals from those studies would contain the true value of the unknown quantity. Alternatives to 95%, such as 90% and 99% confidence intervals, are sometimes used. Wider intervals indicate lower precision; narrow intervals, greater precision.

The Design and Management of Medical Device Clinical Trials: Strategies and Challenges, by Salah Abdel-aleem
Copyright © 2010 John Wiley & Sons, Inc.

Confidence limits The upper and lower boundaries of a confidence interval.

Continuous data Data with a potentially infinite number of possible values within a given range. Height, weight, and blood pressure are examples of continuous variables.

Conformity assessment An activity concerned with determining directly or indirectly that a product complies with established requirements.

Conformity assessment modules Conformity assessment subdivided into individual modules. There are eight modules and variants within the CE marking system.

Contraindication A specific circumstance when the use of certain treatments could be harmful. Sometimes this term is confused with another term namely the use of the product with precaution.

Control group The standard by which experimental observations are evaluated. In many clinical trials, one group of patients will be given an experimental treatment, while the control group is given either a standard treatment for the illness or a placebo.

Cost-effectiveness analysis An economic analysis that view effects in terms of overall health specific to the problem, and describes the costs for some additional health gain.

Declaration of conformity Manufacture's official declaration that a product complies with CE marking.

Directive Pan-European laws pertaining to products and product attributes.

Dose dependent A response to a drug that may be related to the amount received (i.e., the dose). Sometimes trials are done to test the effects of different dosages of the same drug.

Double-blind study A clinical trial design in which neither the participating individuals nor the study staff knows which participants are receiving the experimental treatment and which are receiving a placebo (or another therapy). Double-blind trials are thought to produce objective results, since the expectations of the doctor and the participant about the experimental treatment do not affect the outcome.

Effectiveness The extent to which a specific intervention, when used under ordinary circumstances, does what it is intended to do. For example, if the device is intended for pain relief, it is expected that the device actually relieve pain with evidence demonstrating this effect.

Equivalence trial A trial designed to determine whether the response to two or more treatments differs by an amount that is clinically unimportant. This is usually demonstrated by showing that the true treatment difference is likely to lie between a lower and an upper equivalence level of clinically acceptable differences.

European Economic Area (EEA) The fifteen countries of the EU, plus Iceland, Norway, and Liechtenstein.

European Free Trade Area (EFTA) Iceland, Norway, Liechtenstein, and Switzerland.

European Union Economic union created to enhance political, economic, and social cooperation. Member states include Austria, Belgium, Denmark, Finland, France, Germany, Greece, Ireland, Italy, Luxembourg, Netherlands, Portugal, Spain, Sweden, and the United Kingdom.

European Commission EU government body responsible for proposing and legislating policy.

Essential Requirements The necessary requirements to achieve the objective of the relevant directive. Essential Requirements arise from certain risks, hazards, and/or environmental concerns associated with certain products and/or product attributes.

Food and Drug Administration (FDA) The US Department of Health and Human Services agency responsible for ensuring the safety and effectiveness of all drugs, biologics, and medical devices, including those used in the diagnosis, treatment, and prevention of diseases.

Good clinical practice (GCP) are basically the rules for the design, conduct, performance, monitoring, auditing, recording, analysis, and reporting of clinical trials. They provide assurance that data and results are based on sound scientific and ethical research. They are a broad set of requirements, standards, and recommendations that apply to thousands of highly specific tasks.

Harmonized standards (EN) European product standards published in the *Official Journal* that provide for "presumption of conformity."

Historic control A control person or group for whom data were collected earlier than for the group being studied. There is a large risk of bias in studies that use historic controls due to systematic differences between the comparison groups, due to changes over time in risks, prognosis, health care, and so forth.

Hypothesis A supposition or assumption advanced as a basis for reasoning or argument, or as a guide to experimental investigation.

Technical file (TF)   A documentation file containing the technical basis for a product. All documents used in the CE marking process should be included in this file. This file must be made readily available to a surveillance authority upon request.

Intent-to-treat analysis   Analysis of clinical trial results that includes all data from participants in the groups to which they were randomized even if they never received the treatment or follow the study protocol.

Investigational new drug (IND)   A new drug, antibiotic drug, or biological drug that is used in a clinical investigation. It also includes a biological product used in vitro for diagnostic purposes.

Masked   The knowledge of intervention assignment.

Mean   An average value, calculated by adding all the observations and then dividing by the number of the number of observations.

Meta-analysis   The use of statistical techniques in a systematic review to integrate the results of included studies.

Mutual recognition agreement (MRA)   Agreements to recognize the validity of testing performed outside of the European Union.

New drug application (NDA)   An application submitted by the manufacturer of a drug to the FDA—after clinical trials have been completed—for a license to market the drug for a specified indication.

Noninferiority trial   A trial designed to determine whether the effect of a new treatment is not worse than a standard treatment by more than a prespecified margin.

Notified body   External certification parties designated by European national governments.

Observational study   A study in which the investigators do not seek to intervene, and simply observe the course of events. Changes or differences in one characteristic (e.g., whether or not people received the intervention of interest) are studied in relation to changes or differences in other characteristic(s).

Off-label use   A therapeutic treatment prescribed for conditions other than those approved by the FDA.

Open-label clinical trial   A clinical trial where the investigator and participant are aware of which intervention is being used for which participant (i.e., not blinded).

Per-protocol analysis   An analysis of the subset of participants from a trial who complied with the protocol sufficiently to ensure that their data would be likely to exhibit the effect of treatment. This subset may be defined after considering exposure to treatment, availability of measurements, and absence of major protocol deviations.

p-**Value**   The probability (ranging from zero to one) that the results observed in a study (or results more extreme) could have occurred by chance if in reality the null hypothesis was true. In a meta-analysis the *p*-value for the overall effect assesses the overall statistical significance of the difference between the intervention groups, while the *p*-value for the heterogeneity statistic assesses the statistical significance of differences between the effects observed in each study.

Pharmacokinetics   The processes (in a living organism) of absorption, distribution, metabolism, and excretion of a drug or biologic.

Placebo effect   A physical or emotional change, occurring after a substance is taken or administered, that is not the result of any special property of the substance. The change may be beneficial, reflecting the expectations of the participant, and often the expectations of the person giving the substance.

Protocol   A study plan on which all clinical trials are based. The plan is carefully designed to safeguard the health of the participants as well as answer specific research questions. A protocol describes what types of people may participate in the trial; the schedule of tests, procedures, medications, and dosages; and the length of the study. While in a clinical trial, participants following a protocol are seen regularly by the research staff to monitor their health and to determine the safety and effectiveness of their treatment.

Randomized trial   A study in which participants are randomly (i.e., by chance) assigned to one of two or more treatment arms of a clinical trial. Occasionally placebo is utilized. Randomization minimizes the differences among groups by equally distributing people with particular characteristics among all the trial arms. The researchers do not know which treatment is better.

Safeguard clause   Member states may take all appropriate measures to prohibit or restrict products that pose safety, health, and/or environmental hazards.

Surveillance authorities   Authorities appointed by each participating government to enforce CE marking.

Standards of care   Treatment regimen or medical management based on the state-of-the-art participant care.

Study endpoint   A primary or secondary outcome used to judge the effectiveness of a treatment.

Standard deviation (SD)   A measure of the spread or dispersion of a set of observations, calculated as the average difference from the mean value in the sample.

Standard error (SE)   The standard deviation of the sampling distribution of a statistic. Measurements taken from a sample of the population will vary from sample to sample. The standard error is a measure of the variation in the sample statistic over all possible samples of the same size. The standard error decreases as the sample size increases.

Statistically significant   A result that is unlikely to have happened by chance. The usual threshold for this judgment is that the results, or more extreme results, would occur by chance with a probability of less than 0.05 if the null hypothesis was true. Statistical tests produce a p-value used to assess this.

Stratification   The process by which groups are separated into mutually exclusive subgroups of the population that share a characteristic: for example, age group, sex, or socioeconomic status. It is possible to compare these different strata to try and see if the effects of a treatment differ between the subgroups. *See also* Subgroup analysis.

Subgroup analysis   An analysis in which the intervention effect is evaluated in a defined subset of the participants in a trial, or in complementary subsets, such as by sex or in age categories. Trial sizes are generally too small for subgroup analyses to have adequate statistical power.

Surrogate endpoints   Often physiological or biochemical markers that can be relatively quickly and easily measured, and that are taken as being predictive of important clinical outcomes. Surrogate endpoints are often used when observation of clinical outcomes requires long follow-up. For example, blood pressure is not directly important to patients, but it may be used as an outcome in clinical trials because it is a risk factor for stroke and heart attacks.

***t*-Test**   A statistical hypothesis test derived from the t distribution. It is used to compare continuous data in two groups (also called Student's t-test).

Two-tailed *t*-test   A hypothesis test where the values for which we can reject the null hypothesis are located entirely in both tails of the probability distribution. Testing whether one treatment is either better or worse than another (rather than testing whether one treatment is only better than another) would be a two-tailed test (also called two-sided test).

REFERENCES

1. Altman DG, Schulz KF, Moher D, et al., for the CONSORT group. The revised CONSORT statement for reporting randomised trials: explanation and elaboration. Ann Intern Med 2001;134:663–94.
2. Kirby A, Gebski V, Keech A. Determining the sample size in a clinical trial. Med J Aust 2002;176:256–7.
3. Gebski V, Beller E, Keech AC. Randomised controlled trials, the elements of a good study. Med J Aust 2001;175:272–4.
4. Woodward M. Epidemiology: study design and data analysis. Boca Raton: Chapman and Hall/CRC Press, 1999.
5. Simes RJ, Greatorex V, Gebski VJ. Practical approaches to minimise problems with missing quality of life data. Stat Med 1998;17:725–37.
6. Hollander M, Wolf D. Nonparametric statistical methods, 2nd ed. New York: Wiley, 1999.
7. Martin G. Munchausen's statistical grid, which makes all trials significant. Lancet 1984;ii:1457.
8. Wittes J. On changing a long-term trial midstream. Stat Med 2002;27:2789–95.
9. Preliminary report: effect of encainide and flecainide on mortality in a randomized trial of arrhythmia suppression after myocardial infarction. The Cardiac Arrhythmia Suppression Trial (CAST) Investigators. N Engl J Med 1989;321(6):406–12.
10. Gayet J-L. The OPTIMAAL trial: losartan or captopril after acute myocardial infarction. Lancet 2002;360:1884–5.
11. Stone GW, McLaurin BT, David A, Cox DA, et al. Bivalirudin for patients with acute coronary syndromes. N Engl J Med 2006;355:2203–16.
12. Snappin SM. Alternatives for discounting in the analysis of noninferiority trials. J Biopharm Stat 2004;14:263–73.
13. Moliterno DF, Yakubov SJ, DiBattiste PM, et al. Outcomes at 6 months for the direct comparison of tirofiban and abciximab during percutaneous coronary revascularization with stent placement: the TARGET follow-up study. Lancet 2002;360:355–60.

14. Albers GW, Diener HC, Frison L, et al. Ximelagatran vs. warfarin for stroke prevention in patients with nonvalvular atrial fibrillation: a randomized trial. JAMA 2005;293:690–8.

15. Sacco RL, Diener HC, Yusuf S, et al. Aspirin and extended-release dipyridamole versus clopidogrel for recurrent stroke. N Engl J Med 2008;359: 1238–51.

16. Schweickert W, Hall J. Informed consent in the intensive care unit: ensuring understanding in a complex environment. Curr Opin Crit Care 2005; 11(6):624–8.

17. Gammelgaard A. Informed consent in acute myocardial infarction research. J Med Philos 2004;29(4):417–34.

18. George SL. Reducing patient eligibility criteria in cancer clinical trials. J Clin Oncol 1996;14(4):1364–70.

19. Horwitz RI. Complexity and contradiction in clinical trial research. Am J Med 1987;82(3):498–510.

20. Fisher L, Dixon D, Jerson J, et al. Intention to treat in clinical trials. In: Peace K, Statistical issues in drug research and development. New York: Dekker, 1990.

21. Gillings D, Koch G. The application of the principle of intention-to-treat to the analysis of clinical trials. Clinical Research Bulletin. Basle: Santoz Pharma, September 1990.

22. Hollis S, Campbell F. What is meant by intention to treat analysis? Survey of published randomized controlled trials. BMJ 1999;319:670–4.

23. Armitage P. Exclusions, losses to follow-up and withdrawals in clinical trials. In: Shapiro SH, Louis TA, Clinical trials. New York: Dekker, 1983.

24. Bypass Angioplasty Revascularisation Investigation (BARI). Comparison of coronary bypass surgery with angioplasty in patients with multivessel disease. N Engl J Med 1996;335:217–25.

25. Pocock SJ, Assmann SE, Enos LE, Kasten LE. Subgroup analysis, covariate adjustment and baseline comparisons in clinical trial reporting. Stat Med 2000;21:2917–30.

26. Pocock SJ, Hughes MD, Lee RJ. Statistical problems in reporting of clinical trials: a survey of three medical journals. N Engl J Med 1987;317:426–32.

27. Yusuf S, Wittes J, Probstfield J, Tyroler HA. Analysis and interpretation of treatment effects in subgroups of patients in randomized clinical trials. JAMA 1991;266:93–8.

28. Parker AB, Naylor CD. Subgroups, treatment effects and baseline risks: some lessons from major cardiovascular trials. Am Heart J 2000;139: 952–61.

29. Assmann SF, Pocock SJ, Enos LE, Kasten LE. Subgroup analysis and other mis(uses) of baseline data in clinical trials. Lancet 2000;255:1064–9.

30. Burgess DC, Gebski VJ, Keech AC. Baseline data in clinical trials. Med J Aust 2002;179:105–7.

31. Brookes ST, Whitley E, Peters TJ, et al. Subgroup analyses in randomised controlled trials: quantifying the risks of false positives and false negatives. Health Technol Assess 2001;5:1–56.

32. Lee KL. Clinical judgement and statistics. Lessons from a simulated randomized trial in coronary artery disease. Circulation 1980;61:508–15.

33. ISIS-2 Collaborative Group Randomized trial of IV streptokinase, oral aspirin, both, or neither among 17 187 cases of suspected acute myocardial infarction. Lancet 1988;2:349–60.

34. Hoffman SN, TenBrook JA, Wolf MP, et al. A meta-analysis of randomized controlled trials comparing coronary artery bypass graft with percutaneous transluminal coronary angioplasty: one- to eight-year outcomes. J Am Coll Cardiol 2003;41:1293–304.

35. Niles NW, McGrath PD, Malenka D, et al. Survival of patients with diabetes and multivessel coronary artery disease after surgical or percutaneous coronary revascularization: results of a large regional prospective study. Northern New England Cardiovascular Disease Study Group. J Am Coll Cardiol 2001;37:1008–15.

36. Peto R. Clinical trials. In: Price P, Sikara K, Treatment of cancer, 3rd ed. London: Chapman and Hall, 1995:1039–44.

37. Coates AS, Goldhirsch A, Gelber RD. Overhauling the breast cancer overview: are subsets subversive? Lancet Oncol 2002;3:525–6.

38. Friedman LM, Furberg CD, DeMets DL. Fundamentals of clinical trials, 3rd ed. New York: Springer, 1998:289–93.

39. Hahn S. Assessing the potential for bias in meta-analysis due to selective reporting of subgroup analyses within studies. Stat Med 2000;19:3325–36.

40. Altman DG, Bland JM. Interaction revisited: the difference between two estimates. BMJ 2003;326:219.

41. Frasure-Smith N, Lesperance F, Prince RH, et al. Randomised trial of home-based psychosocial nursing intervention for patients recovering from myocardial infarction. Lancet 1997;350:473–9.

42. Rathore SS, Wang Y, Krumholz HM. Sex-based differences in the effect of digoxin for the treatment of heart failure. N Engl J Med 2002;347:1403–11.

43. Altman DG. Within trial variation—a false trail? J Clin Epidemiol 1998;51:301–3.

44. Hoffman SN, TenBrook JA, Wolf MP, et al. A meta-analysis of randomized controlled trials comparing coronary artery bypass graft with percutaneous transluminal coronary angioplasty: one- to eight-year outcomes. J Am Coll Cardiol 2003;41:1293–304.

45. David I Cook, Val J Gebski, Anthony C Keech. Subgroup analysis in clinical trials. MJA 2 2004;180(6):289–91.

46. Chatfield C, Collins AJ. Introduction to Multivariate Analysis. Chapman and Hall/CRC, 1981.

47. Auleley G-R, Giraudeau B, Baron G, Maillefert J-F, Dougados M, Ravaud P. The methods for handling missing data in clinical trials influence sample size requirements. J Clini Epidemiol 2004;57(5):447–53.

48. Grunkemeier GL, Jin R, Starr A. Prosthetic heart valves: objective performance criteria versus randomized clinical trial. Ann Thorac Surg 2006; 82(3):776–80.

49. Chen E, Sapirstein W, Ahn C, Swain J, Zuckerman B. FDA perspective on clinical trial design for cardiovascular devices. Ann Thorac Surg 2006; 82(3):773–5.

50. Zuckerman BD, Muni NI. Cardiovascular device development: an FDA perspective. Am J Ther 2005;12(2):176–8.

51. Prostanoids for chronic critical leg ischemia. A randomized, controlled, open-label trial with prostaglandin E1. The ICAI Study Group. Ischemia Cronica degli Arti Inferiori. Ann Intern Med 1999;130:412–21.

52. Summary of Safety and Effectiveness of HeratMate II: http://www.fda.gov/cdrh/pdf6/p060040.html.

53. Alleged abuse of research grant money lead to false claims settlement. Report on Medicare Compliance. May 25, 2000.

54. "At Your Own Risk" article on research abuses. Time Magazine, April 22, 2002.

55. Leonard Caputo, MD. Warning letter. CDER issued June 11, 2002.

56. PMA application: P970029 Eclipse Surgical Technologies, Inc. TMR Holmium Laser System.

57. ACCULINK™ and RX ACCULINK™ Carotid Stent System. Summary of Safety and Effectiveness Data.

58. North American Symptomatic Carotid Endarterectomy Trial. Methods, patient characteristics, and progress. Stroke 1991;22(6):711–20.

59. Barnett HJ, Taylor DW, Eliasziw M, Fox AJ, Ferguson GG, Haynes RB, Rankin RN, Clagett GP, Hachinski VC, Sackett DL, Thorpe KE, Meldrum HE. Benefit of carotid endarterectomy in patients with symptomatic moderate or severe stenosis. North American Symptomatic Carotid Endarterectomy Trial Collaborators. N Engl J Med 1998;339(20):1415–25.

60. Endarterectomy for asymptomatic carotid artery stenosis. Executive Committee for the Asymptomatic Carotid Atherosclerosis Study. JAMA 1995;273(18):1421–8.

61. Yadav JS, Wholey MH, Kuntz RE, Fayad P, Katzen BT, Mishkel GJ, Bajwa TK, Whitlow P, Strickman NE, Jaff MR, Popma JJ, Snead DB, Cutlip DE, Firth BG, Ouriel K; Stenting and Angioplasty with Protection in Patients at High Risk for Endarterectomy Investigators. Protected carotid-artery stenting versus endarterectomy in high-risk patients. N Engl J Med 2004;351(15):1493–501.

62. XIENCE V™ (Everolimus Eluting Coronary Stent System). FDA summary of safety and effectiveness. Washington, DC: GPO, 2008.

The Design and Management of Medical Device Clinical Trials: Strategies and Challenges, by Salah Abdel-aleem
Copyright © 2010 John Wiley & Sons, Inc.